The Musculoskeletal System

Endorsed by
St George's, University of London

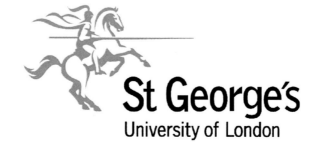

St George's
University of London

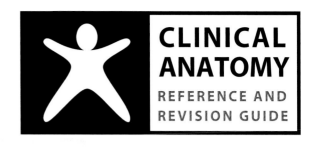

The Musculoskeletal System

Edited by

Philip James Adds, BSc (Hons), MSc, FIBMS
St George's, University of London, London, UK

and

Somayyeh Shahsavari, BSc (Hons), MSc
St George's, University of London, London, UK

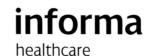

First published in 2012 by Informa Healthcare, Telephone House, 69-77 Paul Street, London EC2A 4LQ, UK.

Simultaneously published in the USA by Informa Healthcare, 52 Vanderbilt Avenue, 7th Floor, New York, NY 10017, USA.

Informa Healthcare is a trading division of Informa UK Ltd. Registered Office: 37–41 Mortimer Street, London W1T 3JH, UK. Registered in England and Wales number 1072954.

A CIP record for this book is available from the British Library.

ISBN-13: 9781841848754

Orders may be sent to: Informa Healthcare, Sheepen Place, Colchester, Essex CO3 3LP, UK
Telephone: +44 (0)20 7017 5540
Email: CSDhealthcarebooks@informa.com
Website: http://informahealthcarebooks.com/

Library of Congress Cataloging-in-Publication Data

The musculoskeletal system / edited by Philip James Adds, Somayyeh Shahsavari ; endorsed by St. George's University of London.
    p. ; cm.
   Includes bibliographical references and index.
   Summary: "The Musculoskeletal System is an anatomy reference and revision guide, combining detailed illustrations with a strong clinical focus, to allow an easier correlation between anatomy and practice. Illustrated with over 100 clinical images and hand-drawn illustrations, and separated in manageable sections by anatomical area, this book provides a compact and complete account of the body's complex system of bones and muscles whilst also considering joints and ligaments, and nerve innervation"--Provided by publisher.
   ISBN 978-1-84184-875-4 (pbk. : alk. paper)
   I. Adds, Philip James. II. Shahsavari, Somayyeh. III. St. George's Hospital (London, England). Medical School.
   [DNLM: 1. Musculoskeletal System--anatomy & histology.]
   LC classification not assigned
   616.7--dc23

                                                                                                    2011029768

For corporate sales please contact: CorporateBooksIHC@informa.com
For foreign rights please contact: RightsIHC@informa.com
For reprint permissions please contact: PermissionsIHC@informa.com

Typeset by Exeter Premedia Services Private Ltd., Chennai, India
Printed and bound in the United Kingdom

Dedication

To my students, past, present and future.

Philip James Adds

I dedicate this book to my incredible family, for their unconditional love and support through the years and for always believing in me. I owe them all that I am and all that I have achieved, especially my parents who have been my inspiration and hope through difficult times. They have taught me to follow my dreams, realise my strengths and conquer my weaknesses. I am forever indebted to them.

Somayyeh Shahsavari

Contents

For the section *Online features*, please visit www.informahealthcare.com

Contributors

Philip James Adds
Division of Biomedical Sciences (Anatomy), St George's, University of London, London, UK

Somayyeh Shahsavari
St George's, University of London, London, UK

Shalina Mitchell
St George's, University of London, London, UK

Harriette Spencer
St George's, University of London, London, UK

Jonathan Warren (our illustrator)
London, UK

Foreword

It gives me great pleasure to be able to write this foreword to what I feel is going to be an important and successful contribution to the clinical anatomy library. I am pleased for several reasons. First and foremost because this is a book written by medical students for medical students. As many medical students will probably agree it is generally much easier to learn from one's peer or near-peer than from one's teacher. Indeed, in the spirit of the Hippocratic oath, there is nothing more noble than to learn from those ahead of us and teach those behind us.

Another reason why I am pleased to write this foreword is that the information presented herein is concise and covers relevant parts of the musculoskeletal anatomy curriculum. There are few greater challenges to medical students than learning human anatomy. The vast array of anatomy reference texts coupled with the current controversies over the place of anatomy in medical curricula does very little to ameliorate this. What textbooks should one read? Should one spend more or less time in the dissecting room? How much time should one spend learning anatomy as opposed to the other medical and clinical sciences? The dilemmas of a medical student abound. This textbook does not add to the confusion but instead presents the relevant information in a way that will appeal to scores of undergraduate medical students. In my opinion the inclusion of clearly tabulated factual information coupled with high quality photographs and colouring images is a particular strength of this textbook.

I have no doubt that this textbook will receive the warm and sustained reception that it so richly deserves.

Peter Bazira
Clinical Senior Lecturer, Hull York Medical School
Formerly Head of Anatomy, St. George's, University of London
London, UK

Acknowledgements

We would like to express our heartfelt gratitude to a number of people without whose support, dedication and tremendous hard work it would not have been possible to complete this book:

Miss Parita Patel, managing editor at Informa Healthcare, who gave us the opportunity to realise our vision for this book. We thank her for her patience, guidance and continuous support throughout this project and for her kind manner and encouraging advice.

We are greatly obliged to Miss Shalina Mitchell and Miss Harriette Spencer, the two incredibly dedicated, hardworking and inspiring contributing authors who have managed to produce exceptionally high quality work alongside studying for their medical degree. It has been a great honour and an enjoyable experience to work with such enthusiastic and committed individuals.

Our illustrator, Mr Jonathan Warren has been a key figure in producing this book. Without his astounding talent and undeniable commitment, it would have been impossible to complete this work. He is a tremendously gifted individual whose humble manner and team work ability has proven vital in the success of this project.

We thank Dr Alan Grundy, consultant radiologist at St George's NHS Trust for his contribution to our "clinical scenarios" chapter, his expert advice and radiological images.

We also wish to express our sincere gratitude to Professor Vishy Mahadevan, Professor of Surgical Anatomy and the Barbers' Company Reader in Anatomy at the Royal College of Surgeons of England, for allowing us to use images of Royal College specimens.

We are greatly indebted to the incredibly generous men and women who donated their bodies to science and gave us the opportunity to expand our knowledge of anatomy and provided us with the most powerful tool in ensuring the continuation of medical training and education.

The editors
P.A.
S.S.

Online features

The online features section is available for viewing at our website:
http://www.informahealthcare.com

To access the features, you will need to first register at our website, where upon completion of the registration process, you will have the necessary login details. If you have previously registered, there is no need to register again.

After you have completed the registration procedure, please type the following link in your Web browser:
http://informahealthcare.com/onlinefeatures/9781841848761

The opening page will request your login details, and after signing in, the material will be available for viewing.

1 Introduction

Somayyeh Shahsavari

The proper study of mankind is man.
—Alexander Pope, *An Essay on Man* (1733)

You are reading this book either as a student of human sciences or as a junior professional in the field; whatever your rank or status on this long and endless ladder of knowledge, you are reading this because you have recognised the importance of understanding the structural map of our existence that is anatomy.

Anatomy is divided into gross and microscopic anatomy. Gross anatomy is visual science; it is what you can see by using the naked eye and nothing more. It is a map that enables you to understand yourself, explore how you function and locate malfunctions that threaten your very existence. Most importantly in the context of this book, however, gross anatomy is the bane of our existence as faithful students of science.

I remember very clearly my first day in the dissection room as a first-year medical student. You could smell the fear and the stress that this cold room had inflicted upon all of us—the fear and stress of miserably failing the end of year anatomy exam. It really did overpower the smell of cadavers.

This book is the result of that first day experience. It is a comprehensive revision and reference guide for those who have studied anatomy through dissection, books, lectures and clinical/surgical experiences. It aims to provide all you need to know about the musculoskeletal system—every bone, every muscle, every joint and every ligament, along with comprehensive clinical photos and illustrations to help you orientate the human body in your mind. There are numerous clinical scenarios to help you prepare for the most common musculo-skeletal problems encountered and accompanying radiological images to clarify descriptions. The array of typical exam questions as well as the colouring images section will, we hope, ensure complete exam success.

It is important to understand that anatomy is the language of human sciences and whether your career choice lies with medicine, surgery, nursing or psychiatry, anatomy is a language common to all these disciplines. It is vital that you maintain an open mind and an enquiring attitude, if you are to master this universal language and be able to use it to communicate effectively.

My personal experience in medicine so far has taught me that the approach to learning anatomy is very different among students and while there are no right or wrong ways of tackling this huge task, there are methods, tips and suggestions that can help with speed of learning and long-term recall. This book has been put together to provide you with a comprehensive collection of these methods with relevance to the musculoskeletal system, and allows you to choose which of these methods suit you best.

The first and perhaps the most important tip is to create a study schedule; there are thousands of new facts and unfamiliar names and terms that you must know and you cannot possibly achieve this by random allocation of your time. You must have a schedule that works for you and that you can stick to; it can be as little as half an hour per week to as much as an hour per day; experiment with time management and start early! To help you with this, we have organised each and every bone, muscle, joint and ligament in tabulated format, highlighting all important features, actions, innervations and more. You can choose to learn one or two components of the table per week, known as "chunking".

The next significant tip is learning general "markings". These are terms that are used frequently to describe anatomical features that are seen more than once in different parts of the body, for example, foramina in bones. If you learn the general terms, you can usually work out locations of structures from the names.

Mnemonics are powerful tools but not everyone will find them useful. If you use mnemonics, it is important that you create your own, as you will remember them much better and this will help significantly with long-term recall. Analogies can also be very helpful, for example, the "*sella turcica*" of the sphenoid bone is a saddle-shaped structure (literally "turkish saddle") that the pituitary gland is positioned on; you can remember this by comparing it to a saddle on a horse.

Another important method is visualisation; try to understand the action of the muscles and bones. The dissection room is probably the best place to do this but if you do not have access to one, you can always visualise. Once you can envisage how a muscle or bone moves, you will never forget its action. This book has the proximal and distal attachments of each muscle tabulated for you followed by the actions, so when revising try to imagine the action in relation to attachments.

These are just some of the many useful tips that are available to ensure exam success and long-term recall. You must try to be creative with your learning; think about facts that have stuck with you for years, think about why. How did you come across this fact? Did you see, read or hear about it? Work out how best you remember things and use this as a revision tool! We have provided a "colouring images" section in this book with images that you can label and colour to help you revise. The additional online access provides you with the opportunity to print these images as many times as necessary, so test yourself continuously; practice is the key to success!

2 Upper limb

Harriette Spencer and Somayyeh Shahsavari

> **OBJECTIVES**
> * Bones of the Upper Limb
> * Muscles of the Upper Limb: Attachment, Action and Innervation
> * Joints of the Upper Limb
> * Ligaments of the Upper Limb
> * Clinical Scenarios
> * Key Pointers

The upper extremity is not designed to provide us with structural stability or weight bearing; these characteristics have been minimised in order to enhance mobility and manipulative ability, ranging from high dexterity in the fingers to a wide range of movements at the shoulder. It is important to note that the extent of disability experienced as a result of injury to the upper limb is not directly proportional to the severity of the injury. We are highly dependent upon this part of our anatomy for activities of daily living, hence it is vital that we understand its structure in relation to its function; any treatment post-injury is aimed at reinstating function through repairing the structural damage.

This chapter will allow you to explore all the ways in which the upper limb is supported and the muscle groups that allow a varied amount of movement.

Table 1 Bones of the Arm and Forearm

Bone	Structure	Muscle attachments	Important features
Humerus (ant)	Head	–	Articulates with glenoid fossa of the scapula
	Anatomical neck	–	–
	Surgical neck	–	Distal to the anatomical neck
	Shaft	Coracobrachialis; lateral and medial heads of triceps brachii	–
	Greater tubercle	Supraspinatus; infraspinatus; teres minor	–
	Lesser tubercle	Subscapularis	–
	Bicipital groove (intertubercular sulcus)	Latissimus dorsi; pectoralis major; teres major	–
	Deltoid tuberosity	Deltoid	Continuous with the crest of the greater tuberosity
	Lateral supracondylar ridge	Extensor carpi radialis longus; brachioradialis	Terminates as the lateral epicondyle
	Medial supracondylar ridge	Pronator teres	Terminates as the medial epicondyle
	Lateral epicondyle	Common extensor tendon	–
	Medial epicondyle	Common flexor tendon	–
	Coronoid fossa	–	Lies proximal to the trochlea
	Capitulum	–	Articulates with the radius
	Trochlea	–	Continuous with the capitulum Articulates with the ulna
	Radial fossa	–	–
Humerus (post)	Spiral groove	–	Formed by the radial nerve and profunda brachii artery (runs between medial and lateral heads of triceps)
	Olecranon fossa	–	–
	Surgical neck	–	–
Scapula (ant)	Superior angle	–	–
	Medial border	Levator scapulae; rhomboid minor; rhomboid major; serratus anterior	–
	Inferior angle	Latissimus dorsi; serratus anterior	Easily palpated and marks the seventh rib and the spine of the seventh thoracic vertebrae
	Suprascapular notch	–	Transmits the suprascapular nerve Bridged by the superior transverse scapular (suprascapular) ligament
	Coracoid process	Short head of biceps brachii; pectoralis minor; coracobrachialis	–
	Acromion	Deltoid	Lateral termination of spine of scapula
	Supraglenoid tubercle	Long head of biceps brachii	Located superior to glenoid fossa
	Infraglenoid tubercle	Long head of triceps brachii	Located inferior to glenoid fossa Larger than supraglenoid tubercle
	Glenoid fossa	–	Lateral to coracoid process Articulation for head of humerus
	Subscapular fossa	Subscapularis	–
	Lateral border	Long head of triceps; teres minor; teres major	–
	Spine of the scapula	–	–

(*Continued*)

Table 1 (*Continued*) Bones of the Arm and Forearm

Bone	Structure	Muscle attachments	Important features
Scapula (post)	Spine of scapula	Trapezius; deltoid	–
	Supraspinous fossa	Supraspinatus	Superior to the spine of the scapula
	Infraspinous fossa	Infraspinatus	Inferior to the spine of the scapula
Clavicle	Clavicle	Deltoid; trapezius; sternocleidomastoid; Pectoralis major; subclavius (inferior)	–
	Capsule of acromioclavicular joint	–	–
	Capsule of sternoclavicular joint	–	–
	Conoid tubercle	–	Attachment for the conoid ligament
Radius	Shaft	Flexor digitorum superficialis; flexor pollicis longus; pronator teres; pronator quadratus; supinator	–
	Head	–	Articulates with the capitulum
	Neck	Supinator	–
	Radial tuberosity	Biceps brachii	–
	Styloid process	Brachioradialis	–
Ulna	Shaft	Flexor digitorum profundus; pronator quadratus; extensor pollicis brevis; extensor pollicis longus; extensor indicis	–
	Olecranon	Triceps brachii	–
	Radial notch	–	Articulates with the radius at the proximal radioulnar joint
	Coronoid process	Brachialis; pronator teres (medial head); flexor carpi ulnaris (ulnar head); flexor digitorum superficialis	–
	Styloid process	–	–
	Supinator crest	Supinator	–

Each upper limb consists of a total of 32 bones and these are divided as follows. The shoulder consists of two bones and each arm consists of three; there are eight bones in each wrist and 19 in each hand. The images below highlight the important structures in each bone and the explanations can be found in the table above.

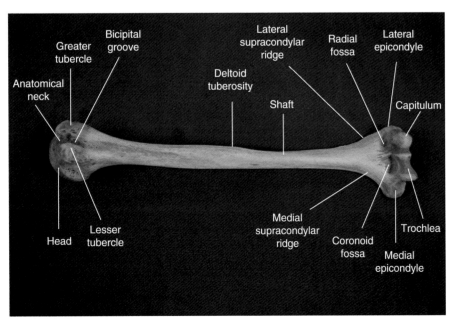

Figure 1a Humerus (Anterior).

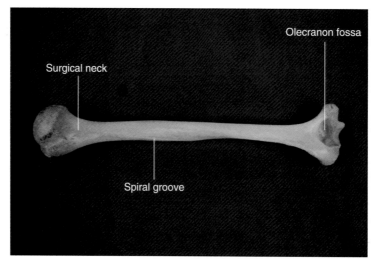

Figure 1b Humerus (Posterior).

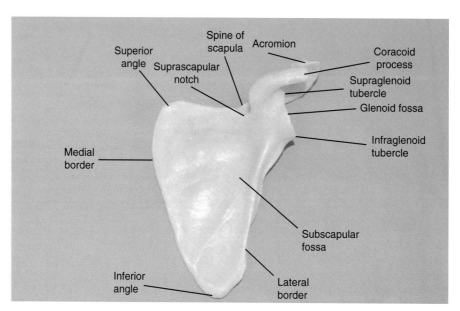

Figure 2a Scapula (Anterior).

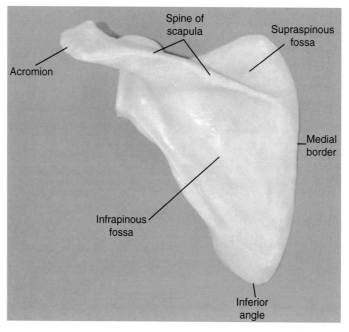

Figure 2b Scapula (Posterior).

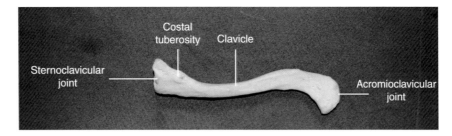

Figure 3 The clavicle; inferior surface.

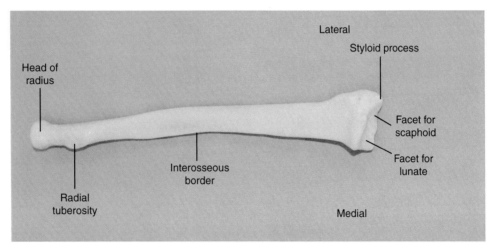

Figure 4a Radius and ulna (posterior).

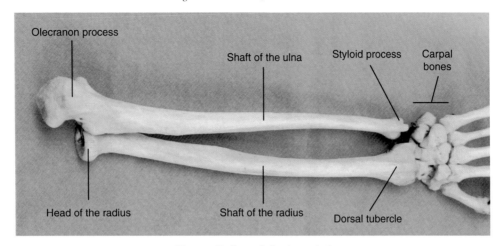

Figure 4b Radius.

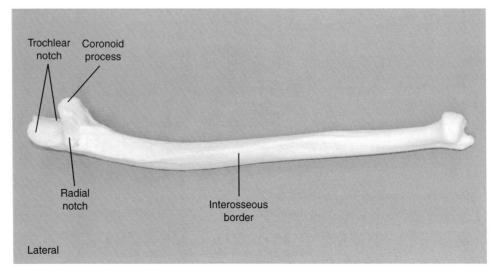

Figure 4c Ulna.

Table 2 Bones of the Hand

Bone	Muscle attachments	Important features
Scaphoid	Abductor pollicis brevis Radial collateral ligament Flexor retinaculum	Tubercle Palpable in the anatomical snuff box
Lunate	–	–
Triquetral	–	Insertion of collateral ligaments of the wrist
Pisiform	Abductor digiti minimi	Sesmoid bone in the tendon of flexor carpi ulnaris Flexor retinaculum attachment
Hamate	Flexor retinaculum Flexor carpi ulnaris Flexor digiti minimi Opponens digiti minimi	–
Capitate	Oblique head of adductor pollicis	Insertion of interosseous ligaments
Trapezoid	–	–
Trapezium	Flexor retinaculum Abductor pollicis brevis Opponens pollicis	–
Metacarpals	Interossei (palmar and dorsal) adductor pollicis Flexor carpi radialis (2nd and 3rd MC) Flexor carpi ulnaris (pisiform and 5th MC) Extensor carpi radialis longus (2nd MC) Extensor carpi radialis brevis (3rd MC) Extensor carpi ulnaris (5th MC) Abductor pollicis longus (1st MC) Opponens pollicis (1st MC)	–
Phalanges	Extensor pollicis longus and brevis Flexor pollicis longus; flexor pollicis brevis; adductor pollicis (1st digit) Flexor digitorum superficialis Extensor digitorum Extensor indicis Extensor digiti minimi Flexor digitorum profundus	–

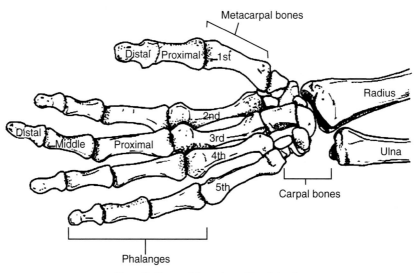

Figure 5a Bones of the wrist and hand sketch.

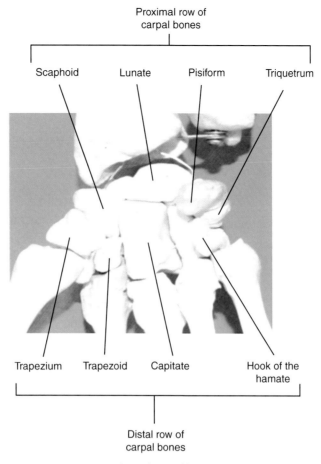

Figure 5b Carpal bones.

The upper limb can be divided into separate functional compartments; the arm has flexor and extensor compartments, as does the forearm. The functional compartments of the hand include the hypothenar and thenar eminences, which along with some of the muscles of the forearm allow fine motor movements of the fingers. Many of the muscles will span at least one joint to both move and support that joint.

The actions of each muscle, along with its attachments and innervation, are detailed in the tables above. The anatomical arrangements are illustrated in the images and sketches below.

Table 3a Muscles of Shoulder

Muscle	Proximal attachment	Distal attachment	Action	Innervation
Trapezius (3 divisions)	Superior nuchal line (occipital bone), nuchal ligament, spinous processes of C7-T12	Lateral third of the clavicle (superior fibres), acromion and spine of the scapula (middle fibres), medial part of spine of the scapula (inferior fibres)	Elevation (superior division) and retraction (middle division) of the scapula Lateral flexion Rotation of scapula Depression (inferior division) of the scapula	Spinal part of the accessory cranial nerve (CNXI), cervical nerves 3 and 4 (proprioception)
Latissimus Dorsi	Spinous processes of thoracic vertebrae 6-12, iliac crest, lower 4 ribs, thoraco-lumbar fascia	Intertubercular sulcus of the humerus (bicipital groove)	Extension and medial rotation Adduction	Thoracodorsal nerve (C6–C8)
Levator Scapulae	Transverse processes of cervical vertebrae 1-4 (C1-4)	Superior angle and superior medial border of the scapula	Rotation of scapula to raise the medial border of the scapula, depressing the glenoid cavity Elevation, lateral flexion of neck	Dorsal scapula nerve (C5)

(*Continued*)

Table 3a (*Continued*) Muscles of Shoulder

Muscle	Proximal attachment	Distal attachment	Action	Innervation
Rhomboid Minor	Spinous processes of cervical vertebrae 7- thoracic 1 (C7-T1)	Medial border of the scapula	Elevation of scapula, scapula rotation during adduction of the upper limb Retraction Helps to hold the scapula to the wall of the thoracic cavity	Dorsal scapular nerve (C5)
Rhomboid Major	Spinous processes of Thoracic vertebrae 2-5 (T2-5)	Medial border of the scapula	Elevation of scapula, scapula rotation during adduction of the upper limb Retraction	Dorsal scapular nerve (C5)
Supraspinatus	Supraspinous fossa of the scapula	Greater tubercle of the humerus	Initiates abduction (first 15°) of the upper limb. Rotator cuff	Suprascapular nerve (C5, C6)
Infraspinatus	Infraspinous fossa of the scapula	Greater tubercle of the humerus	Rotator cuff, lateral rotation of humerus	Suprascapular nerve
Teres Minor	Lateral edge of the scapula	Greater tubercle of the humerus	Rotator cuff, lateral rotation of humerus	Axillary nerve (C5, C6)
Teres major	Lower part of the posterior lateral edge of the scapular	Medial lip of bicipital groove	Adduction of arm Medial rotation and extension of arm	Lower subscapular nerve (C5, C6)
Subscapularis	Medial costal surface of the scapula	Lesser tubercle	Rotator cuff, medial rotation of arm	Upper and lower subscapular nerves (C5, C6)

Table 3b Muscles of the Upper Arm

Muscle	Proximal attachment	Distal attachment	Action	Innervation
Biceps brachii (2 heads)	Supraglenoid tubercle (long head), coracoid process (short head)	Radial tuberosity	Flexion of elbow Supination, weak flexion of shoulder joint	Musculocutaneous nerve (C5-6)
Coracobrachialis	Coracoid process	Half way down the humerus	Weak flexion Adduction and stabilisation of shoulder	Musculocutaneous nerve (C5-6)
Brachialis	Distal half of the shaft of the humerus	Coronoid process of the ulna	Powerful flexion of elbow	Musculoctaneous nerve (C5-6)
Deltoid	Lateral 3rd of the clavicle, acromion, spine of the scapula	Deltoid tuberosity of the humerus	Main abductor of the shoulder Anterior (along with the pec. major) flexion Posterior (along with the lats & teres maj.) extension	Axillary nerve (C5, 6)
Triceps (3 heads)	Infraglenoid tubercle (long head), posterior aspect of the shaft of the humerus, above the radial groove (lateral head) and below the radial groove (medial head)	Olecranon process of the ulna	Extension of elbow Long head: stabilisation of shoulder joint in full abduction	Radial nerve (C7, 8)
Brachioradialis	Lateral supracondylar ridge of the humerus	Radial styloid process	Weak flexion of elbow Rotation of arm from full pronation or supination into the intermediate position	Radial nerve (C5, 6)

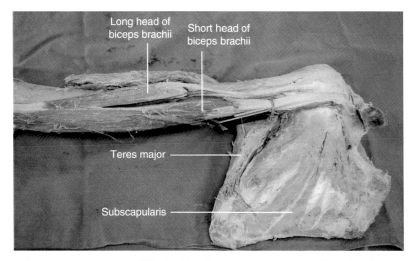

Figure 6a The anterior compartment of the shoulder. The most anterior rotator cuff muscle is the subscapularis.

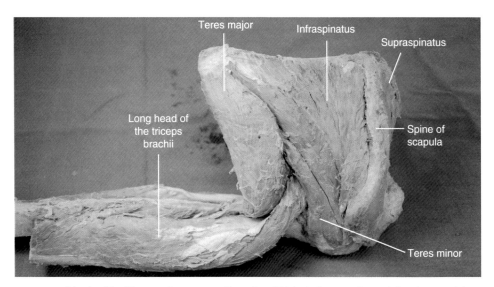

Figure 6b Posterior compartment of the shoulder. The posterior rotator cuff muscles which include supraspinatus, infraspinatus and the teres minor help with the mobility and stability of the glenohumeral joint.

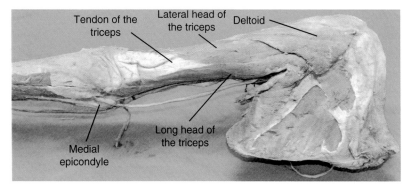

Figure 6c Posterior compartment of the arm.

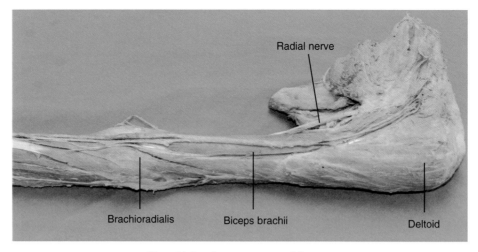

Figure 6d Anterior compartment of the arm.

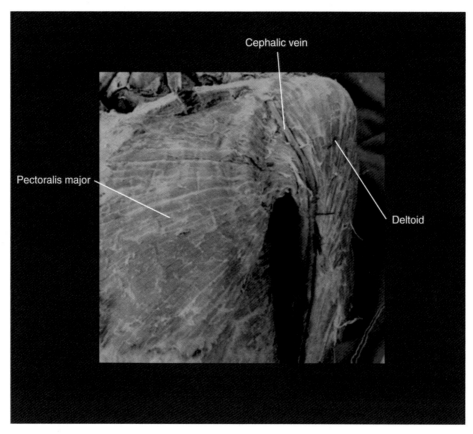

Figure 6e The deltoid and pectoralis major.

Table 4 Muscles of Forearm

Muscle	Proximal attachment	Distal attachment	Action	Innervation
Superficial flexor muscles				
Pronator teres	Common flexor origin (medial epicondyle of humerus), coronoid process	Lateral surface of the radius	Pronation and flexion of forearm	Median nerve (C6, C7)
Flexor carpi radialis	Common flexor origin	2nd and 3rd metacarpals	Flexion and abduction of the wrist Stabilisation of wrist joint during movement of the fingers and thumb	Median nerve (C6, C7)

(*Continued*)

Table 4 (*Continued*) Muscles of Forearm

Muscle	Proximal attachment	Distal attachment	Action	Innervation
Flexor carpi ulnaris (2 heads, humeral and ulnar)	Common flexor origin, medial border of the olecranon	Pisiform, hamate, 5th metacarpal	Flexion and adduction	Ulnar nerve (C7, C8)
Flexor digitorum superficialis (2 heads, humeroulnar and radial)	Common flexor origin, ulnar collateral ligament, coronoid process (humeroulnar), superior portion of anterior radius (radial)	4 tendons to the middle phalanges of the medial 4 digits	Flexion of wrist, metacarpophalangeal & proximal interphalangeal (PIP) joints	Median nerve (C7, C8)
Palmaris longus (absent in approx 13% of arms)	Common flexor origin	Flexor retinaculum, palmar aponeurosis	Weak flexion of wrist, anchors the skin of palm	Median nerve (C7, C8)
Deep flexor muscles				
Flexor digitorum profundus	Shaft of ulnar and interosseous membrane	4 tendons to the distal phalanges of the medial 4 digits	Flexion of distal interphalangeal (DIP) joints	Ulnar nerve (digits 4 & 5) (C8, T1), median nerve (digits 2 & 3) (C8, T1) (anterior interosseous branch)
Flexor pollicis longus	Anterior surface of the radius and interosseous membrane	Distal phalanx of the thumb	Flexion of interphalangeal and metacarpophalangeal (MCP) joint of the thumb	Median nerve (anterior interosseous branch) (C8, T1)
Pronator quadratus	Shaft of the distal part of the ulna	Shaft of the distal part of the radius	Pronation of forearm	Median nerve (anterior interosseous branch) (C8, T1)
Superficial extensor muscles				
Anconeus	Common extensor origin (Lateral epicondyle of the humerus)	Olecranon, proximal ulna	Assists triceps in extension of elbow	Radial nerve (C7, C8)
Extensor carpi ulnaris	Common extensor origin	Base of the 5th metacarpal	Extension and adduction of wrist	Radial nerve (posterior interosseus branch) (C6–C8)
Extensor carpi radialis longus	Common extensor origin, lower third of the supracondylar ridge	Base of the 2nd metacarpal bone	Extension and abduction of wrist	Radial nerve (C6, C7)
Extensor carpi radialis brevis	Common extensor origin	Base of the 3rd metacarpal bone	Extension, abduction	Radial nerve (posterior interosseous) (C6, C7)
Extensor digitorum (communis)	Common extensor origin	Divided into four tendons to the extensor expansions of the medial 4 digits	Extension of fingers and wrist joint	Radial nerve (posterior interosseous nerve) (C6–C8)
Extensor digiti minimi	Common extensor origin	Two tendons to the dorsal expansion of the little finger	Extension of little finger	Radial nerve (posterior interosseous nerve) (C6–C8)
Deep				
Supinator	Common extensor origin, ulna, radial collateral ligament, annular ligament	Lateral surface of the proximal radius	Supination of forearm whilst arm is in any position	Posterior interosseous nerve (C6–C8)
Abductor pollicis longus	Posterior aspect of the ulna, radius and interosseous membrane	Base of the first metacarpal	Abduction, extension and lateral rotation of thumb	Posterior interosseous nerve (C7, C8)

(*Continued*)

Table 4 (*Continued*) Muscles of Forearm

Muscle	Proximal attachment	Distal attachment	Action	Innervation
Extensor pollicis longus	Posterior surface of the middle 3rd of the ulna and interosseous membrane	Distal phalanx of the thumb	Extension of MCP and interphalangeal joints of thumb	Posterior interosseous nerve (C7, C8)
Extensor pollicis brevis	Posterior surface of the radius and interosseous membrane	Base of the proximal phalanx of the thumb	Extension of proximal phalanx of thumb at the MCP joint	Posterior interosseous nerve (C7, C8)
Extensor indicis	Ulna and interosseous membrane	Extensor expansion of 2nd digit	Extension of index finger Assists extension of wrist	Posterior interosseous nerve (C7, C8)

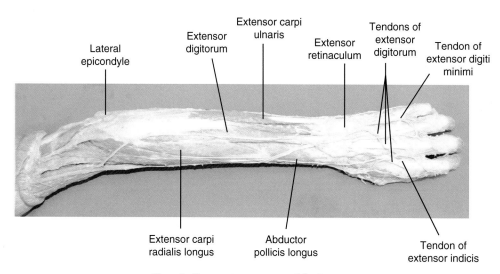

Figure 7a Extensor compartment of the forearm.

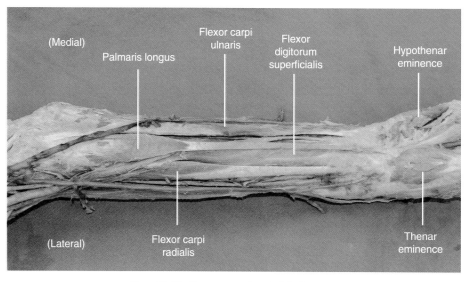

Figure 7b The flexor compartment of the forearm.

Table 5 Muscles of the Hand

Muscle	Proximal attachment	Distal attachment	Action	Innervation
Hypothenar eminence				
Abductor digiti minimi	Pisiform	Proximal phalanx of 5th digit	Abduction of 5th digit	Ulnar nerve (deep branch) (C8, T1)
Flexor digiti minimi	Hamate (hook), flexor retinaculum	Proximal phalanx of 5th digit	Flexion of 5th digit	Ulnar nerve (deep branch) (C8, T1)
Opponens digiti minimi	Hamate (hook), flexor retinaculum	5th metacarpal	Opposition of 5th digit towards the thumb-abduction, flexion and lateral rotation	Ulnar nerve (deep branch) (C8, T1)
Palmaris brevis	Transverse carpal ligament, superficial palmar fascia	Hypothenar skin fascia	Tightens the hypothenar skin	Ulnar nerve (deep branch) (C8, T1)
Thenar eminence				
Abductor pollicis brevis	Scaphoid, trapezium, flexor retinaculum	Base of the proximal phalanx of thumb	Abduction of the carpometacarpal & MCP joints of the thumb	Median nerve (recurrent branch) (C8, T1)
Flexor pollicis brevis (2 heads)	Trapezium, flexor retinaculum (superficial head), carpal canal (trapezoid, capitate) (deep head)	Base of the proximal phalanx & metacarpal bone of thumb via a common tendon containing a sesamoid bone	Flexion of the thumb	Median nerve (recurrent branch) (C8, T1)
Opponens pollicis	Trapezium, flexor retinaculum	1st metacarpal	Opposition of the thumb	Median nerve (recurrent branch) (C8, T1)
Adductor pollicis (oblique and transverse heads)	Capitate, base of 2nd and 3rd metacarpals (oblique head), shaft of 3rd metacarpal (transverse head)	MCP joint of the thumb (on the sesamoid bone)	Adduction	Ulnar nerve (deep branch) (C8, T1)
Deep				
Lumbricals	Tendons of flexor digitorum profundus	Lateral side of extensor expansions (digits 2-5)	Flexion at MCP joints Extension at interphalangeal joints	Median nerve (lateral 2 lumbricals), ulnar nerve (medial 2 lumbricals) (both C8, T1)
Dorsal interossei (4)	Adjacent pairs of metacarpal bones	Base of proximal phalanx/ extensor expansion: <ul><li>1st – lateral side of index finger</li><li>2nd and 3rd – lateral and medial sides of middle finger respectively</li><li>4th – medial side of ring finger</li></ul>	Abduction, (with respect to the axis of the middle finger)	Ulnar nerve (deep branch) (C8, T1)
Palmar interossei (3)	2nd, 4th and 5th metacarpals	Base of proximal phalanx of index, fourth and fifth fingers	Adduction (with respect to the axis of the middle finger)	Ulnar nerve (deep branch) (C8, T1)

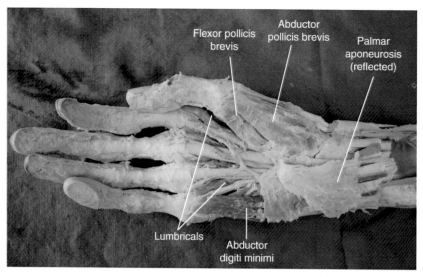

Figure 8a Muscles of the hand (palmar surface).

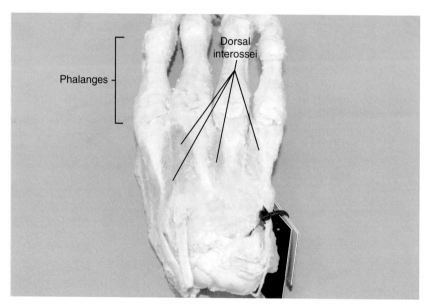

Figure 8b Dorsal interosseous.

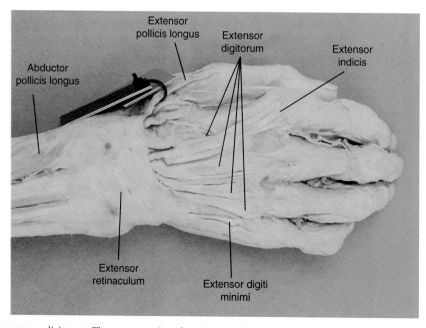

Figure 8c The tendons of the extensor digitorum. The extensor retinaculum is exposed under which run the tendons of extensor digitorum which will form the extensor hoods of the phalanges.

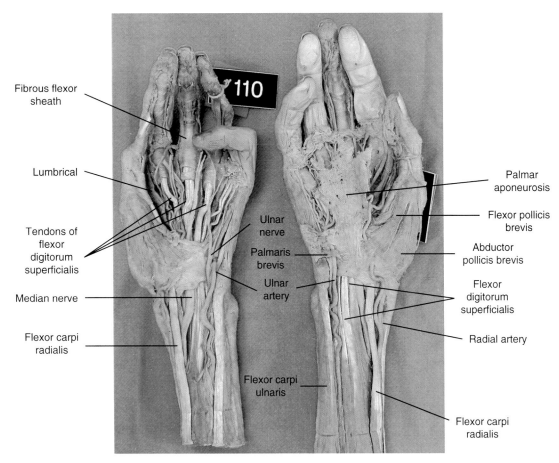

Fibrous flexor
sheath

Lumbrical

Tendons of
flexor
digitorum
superficialis

Median nerve

Flexor carpi
radialis

Ulnar
nerve

Palmaris
brevis

Ulnar
artery

Flexor carpi
ulnaris

Palmar
aponeurosis

Flexor pollicis
brevis

Abductor
pollicis brevis

Flexor
digitorum
superficialis

Radial artery

Flexor carpi
radialis

Figure 8d Features of the hand (palmar surface).

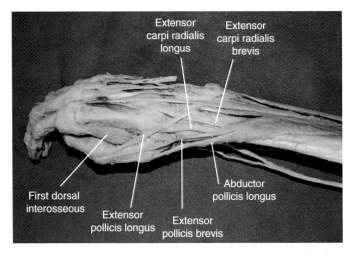

Extensor
carpi radialis
longus

Extensor
carpi radialis
brevis

Abductor
pollicis longus

First dorsal
interosseous

Extensor
pollicis longus

Extensor
pollicis brevis

Figure 8e The anatomical snuff box. This is formed by the tendons of the extensor pollicis longus, extensor pollicis brevis and the abductor pollicis longus. The radial artery runs over the scaphoid in the floor of the snuff box.

The upper limb is connected to the axial skeleton through the connection between the sternum and the clavicle at the sternoclavicular joint and it is the junction of the humerus and scapula at the glenohumeral (shoulder) joint that allows the upper limb such a great range of movement.

The forearm is composed of the radius and the ulna which are connected to the humerus via the elbow joint and also the hand which is composed of the carpal bones, metacarpal bones and the phalanges. The movements between these joints show much greater limitations than those of the glenohumeral but with an increase in stability.

The type and articulations of each joint, along with its action and important features, are detailed in the tables below.

Table 6 Joints of Upper Limb

Joint	Type	Articulations	Action	Important features
Acromioclavicular	Plane (synovial)	Acromion (scapula) to the clavicle (lateral end)	Gliding motion on rotation of the scapula	Ligaments: • Superior and inferior acromioclavicular ligaments • Coracoclavicular ligament (conoid and trapezoid parts) Innervation: • Suprascapular nerve
Carpometacarpal joints	Saddle	Trapezium First metacarpal bone	Flexion Extension Abduction Adduction Opposition (1st digit only)	Ligaments: • Dorsal • Palmar • Interosseous
	Plane (synovial)	Base of metacarpal bones Distal row of carpal bones	Slight gliding movement only	
Distal interphalangeal (DIPS)	Hinge (synovial)	Distal phalanx Middle phalanx	Flexion Extension	Ligaments: • Collateral ligaments
Distal radio-ulnar	Pivot (synovial)	Head of ulna Ulnar notch of radius Articular disc	Pronation Supination	Ligaments: • Anterior ligament • Posterior ligament Innervation: • Anterior interosseous nerve
Elbow	Hinge (synovial)	Trochlea and capitulum of the humerus Trochlear notch of ulna Head of radius	Flexion Extension	Ligaments: • Lateral collateral ligament • Medial collateral ligament Innervation: • Median nerve • Ulnar nerve • Musculocutaneous nerve • Radial nerve
Glenohumeral (Shoulder)	Ball and socket (synovial)	Head of the humerus The glenoid cavity of the scapula	Wide range of movement (with minimal stability) • Flexion • Extension • Abduction • Adduction • Lateral rotation • Medial rotation • Circumduction	Ligaments: • Glenohumeral ligaments • Transverse humeral ligament • Coracohumeral ligament • Coracoacromial ligament Innervation: • Axillary nerve • Suprascapular nerve

(*Continued*)

Table 6 (*Continued*) Joints of Upper Limb

Joint	Type	Articulations	Action	Important features
Intercarpal	Plane (synovial)	Between the individual bones and between the proximal and distal rows of carpal bones	Gliding movement	Ligaments: • Dorsal and palmar ligaments • Interosseous ligaments Innervation: • Anterior interosseous nerve • Deep branch of radial nerve • Deep branch of ulnar nerve
Metocarpophalangeal	Condyloid	Proximal phalanges Head of metacarpals	Flexion Extension Abduction Adduction	Ligaments: • Palmar ligament • Deep transverse metacarpal ligaments • Collateral ligaments
Proximal Interphalangeal (PIPS)	Hinge (synovial)	Middle phalanx Proximal phalanx	Flexion Extension	Ligaments: • Collateral ligaments Innervation: • Palmar digital nerves
Proximal radio-ulnar	Pivot (synovial)	Head of radius Annular ligament Radial notch of the ulna	Pronation Supination	Ligaments: • Annular ligament Innervation: • Median nerve • Ulnar nerve • Musculocutaneous nerve • Radial nerve
Radiocarpal joint	Ellipsoid (synovial)	Distal radius plus articular disc Scaphoid Lunate Triquetral bone	Flexion Extension Abduction (radial deviation) Adduction (ulnar deviation)	Ligaments: • Anterior ligament • Posterior ligament • Ulnar collateral ligament • Radial collateral ligament Innervation: • Anterior interosseous nerve • Deep branch of radial nerve
Sternoclavicular	Saddle, with an articular disc (synovial) Functionally ball and socket	First costal cartilage Clavicle Manubrium of sternum	Movement of the clavicle	Ligaments: • Sternoclavicular ligament • Costoclavicular ligament • Interclavicular ligament Innervation: • Supraclavicular nerve

A ligament is an attachment between either two bones or bone and cartilage, hence forming a joint and providing a limited range of movements at that joint. With this limitation comes greater alignment of bones and more controlled and precise movements.

Exercises that focus on flexibility help increase the range of motion at the joints, not by stretching the ligaments but by increasing the length and flexibility of muscles. Excessive strain and direct trauma can cause ligament injury and repetitive injuries can lead to weakening of the joint involved.

Ligaments also have minimal blood supply as they are designed to endure high levels of stress and/or load-bearing on daily basis; as a result injuries are slow to heal and may require surgical intervention and physiotherapy.

Table 7 Ligaments of the Upper Limb

Ligament	Attachment	Function
Glenohumeral joint		
Conoid (coracoclavicular)	Coracoid process (medial to the trapezoid) Conoid tubercle of the inferior surface of the clavicle	Controls anterior posterior stability of the joint between the coracoid process and the clavicle
Coracoacromial	Coracoid process Acromion	Reinforces the glenohumeral joint superiorly
Coracohumeral	Coracoid process Greater tubercle of humerus	Reinforces anterior part of glenohumeral joint capsule
Glenohumeral (inferior)	Glenoid labrum Anatomical neck of humerus	Additional restraint to the superior glenohumeral ligament especially when the arm is abducted at 90°
Glenohumeral (middle)	Glenoid labrum, inferior to the superior glenohumeral ligament Medial to the lesser tubercle of the humerus	Additional restraint to the superior glenohumeral ligament especially when the arm is abducted at 45°
Glenohumeral (superior)	From upper part of the glenoid labrum Superior to the lesser tubercle of the humerus	A restraint to prevent anterior and posterior subluxation whilst the arm is adducting
Superior transverse scapular	Coracoid process Medial portion of scapular notch	Creates the scapular notch through which the suprascapular nerve runs
Trapezoid (coracoclavicular)	Coracoid process (lateral to the conoid) Inferior surface of the clavicle	Controls anterior-posterior stability of the joint between the coracoid process and the clavicle
Elbow joint		
Annular	Margins of the radial notch of the ulna. Encloses the head of the radius Radius	Keeps the head of the radius in contact with the radial notch of the ulnar stabilising the proximal radio-ulnar joint
Radial collateral	Lateral epicondyle of the humerus Annular ligament	Strengthens the side walls of the elbow joint capsule stabiliser during flexion
Ulnar collateral	Medial epicondyle Coronoid process Olecranon	Stabilises medial sides of elbow joint The ligament has three parts: Anterior oblique (AO) Posterior oblique (PO) Small transverse (ST)
Hand		
Deep transverse metacarpal ligament	Between the heads of the metacarpal bones	Restraint to the movement of the metacarpal bones
Dorsal radiocarpal	Styloid process of radius Dorsal surface of scaphoid, lunate and triquetrum	Limits radial deviation of the wrist
Extensor retinaculum	Styloid process of the radius Pisiform Triquetrum	Prevents bowstringing of the extensor tendons
Flexor retinaculum	Scaphoid tubercle Trapezium Pisiform Hook of hamate	Palmaris brevis and longus insert into it The median nerve passes deep to it in the carpal tunnel
Interosseous intercarpal	Carpal bones	Limit movement of the carpal bones
Lateral collateral	Lateral side of the head of the metacarpal bone Base of the phalanx	Limit movement at the metacarpophalangeal joint whilst in flexion

(Continued)

Table 7 (*Continued*) Ligaments of the Upper Limb

Ligament	Attachment	Function
Medial collateral	Medial side of the head of the metacarpal bone Base of the phalanx	Limits movement at the metacarpophalangeal joint whilst in flexion
Palmar	Proximal phalanx Metacarpal bones	Limits movement at the metacarpophalangeal joint
Palmar ulnocarpal	Styloid process of radius Lunate Triquetrum	Limits extension of the wrist
Palmar radiocarpal	Styloid process of ulnar Proximal carpal bones	Limits radial deviation of the wrist
Ulna collateral	Styloid process of ulna Triquetrum	Supports the radiocarpal joint
Radial collateral	Styloid process of radius Scaphoid bone	Supports the radiocarpal joint

CLINICAL SCENARIOS

Colles Fracture

A 72-year-old female presents to A&E with confusion, pain in the right arm and hand and inability to move her right wrist. You discover that she has had a fall outside the supermarket, on the concrete floor of the entrance. She describes feeling dizzy, losing her balance and falling backwards on her outstretched arm and open palm. Study the X-ray below (Fig. 9).

Typical Findings
- A distal radius fracture usually seen in the elderly with osteoporosis.
- A clear dorsal slanting of the hand: "dinner fork" appearance.
- Fracture is about 4 cm proximal to the radio-carpal joint.
- Shortened radius.
- Radial deviation.
- The ulnar styloid process may also be fractured.

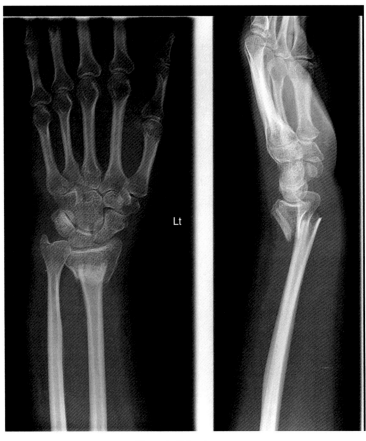

Figure 9 Colles fracture.

Smith's Fracture

You are an F2 doctor on your orthopaedic surgery rotation. You have been called to see a 45-year-old man who has had a fall from a height of about 1.5 m and landed on his front with his arm extended and his hand "twisted inwards". He is in pain and cannot move his left wrist. You order an X-ray (Fig. 10).

Typical Findings

- Can be caused by a high-impact blow to the dorsum of the forearm or by a fall on the wrist in flexed position.
- Also known as the "garden spade" deformity.
- The wrist clearly sits anteriorly compared to its normal anatomical position.

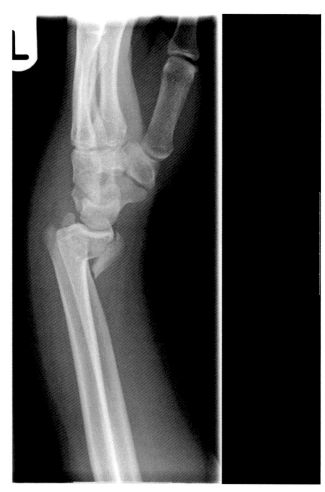

Figure 10 Smith's fracture.

Scaphoid Fracture

A 13-year-old boy has been referred to your orthopaedic clinic by his GP, following an incident at school 2 weeks ago, which involved a direct blow to the dorsum of his hand and wrist. He tells you that the deep and dull pain as a result of the "sprain" has not settled and he is finding it increasingly difficult to "grip stuff". The area appears swollen and painful to touch, particularly in the snuff box region and the Watson test also elicits pain (moving the wrist back and forth with the thumb on the scaphoid bone). The X-ray ordered by the GP revealed an incomplete scaphoid fracture (Fig. 11).

Typical Findings
- Roughly 11% of scaphoid fractures are incomplete.
- Complete fractures can be classified as tubercle, transverse waist and proximal pole fractures.
- The X-ray may not reveal a fracture if carried out immediately and a 10-day repeat X-ray may be required.
- The position of the bone and its size make it difficult to detect a fracture.

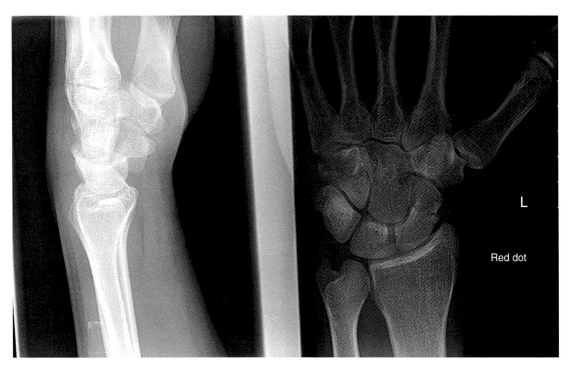

Figure 11 Scaphoid fracture.

Barton's Fracture

A 35-year-old female presents to A&E having fallen off her bicycle when trying to avoid a collision with a car. She describes hitting the concrete and landing on the right side of her body and remembers trying to "cushion her fall" with her right arm stretched out; she landed on her wrist. By carrying out a full examination and in line with her other injuries, you decide that the fall was of a high impact and order an X-ray (Fig. 12).

Typical Findings
- This is an intra-articular radius fracture with dorsal or palmar subluxation (dislocation) of the carpal bones.

- There are two types: dorsal and palmar; the latter is more common.
- The mechanism of this injury is quite similar to that of Smith's fracture but caused by higher impact and greater loading on the wrist.
- The X-ray interpretation is difficult for inexperienced junior doctors due to its many similarities with Smith's fracture. However, an experienced eye can see a degree of carpal displacement, which then confirms the diagnosis.

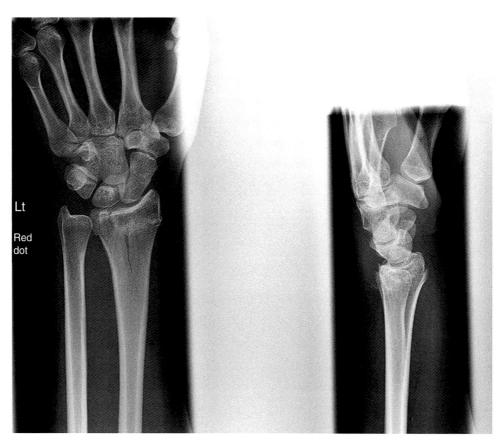

Figure 12 Barton's Fracture.

Greenstick Fracture

An anxious mother has brought her 6-year-old daughter to A&E after receiving a call about an accidental fall in the playground. The child appears in pain and is quite distressed and has her right arm supported by her mother. On examination, the arm appears normal in shape and size and there are no obvious signs of fracture but the pain intensifies on palpation, particularly on the dorsal forearm, roughly 3–4 cm proximal to the radio-carpal joint. You order X-rays of both arms (Fig. 13), injured arm only shown.

Typical Findings
- This is a typical fracture seen in children under 12 years of age.
- An incomplete break due to the bones being softer than in adults.
- It is due to the incomplete fracture that the shape and contour of the site of fracture may remain unchanged.
- It is common for physicians to X-ray the uninjured arm also, for comparison purposes.

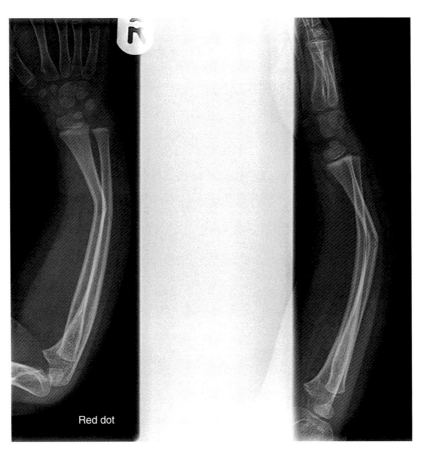

Red dot

Figure 13 Greenstick fracture.

Elbow Fractures/Injuries

Olecranon Fracture

A 70-year-old male has been brought to A&E after a fall at home. He remembers getting up from his chair, losing his balance and falling "quite suddenly" to the ground. He explains that he tried to cushion the fall with his left arm. On examination, the entire arm is painful to touch and there is particular tenderness around the elbow region along with effusion that you suspect is haemorrhagic. The patient is also unable to extend his elbow by himself and confirms your suspicion of triceps muscle involvement. You request an X-ray.

Typical Findings
- The semiflexed and slightly supinated arm is the common position that causes this type of fracture, on impact.
- On hitting the ground, triceps and brachialis muscles tense to cushion the fall and snap the olecranon in the process.
- A fall in the elderly is the most common cause of this fracture, followed by direct blow to the elbow.
- Most common X-ray finding is an oblique fracture at the base of the olecranon.

Coronoid Process Fracture

You have been called to see an 8-year-old boy in A&E, who has been brought in by his mother following a fall in the garden. He looks clearly distressed and you immediately notice a deformed right elbow. You manage to gather from a combination of direct and collateral history that he has fallen on an outstretched arm while chasing the family pet cat. On examination, there are limited extension, flexion and rotation movements, as well as clear displacement and crepitations. The neurological and vascular exams are unremarkable. You suspect a case of terrible triad and request an X-ray.

Typical Findings
- Coronoid fractures are common in children and occur mainly due to a fall on an outstretched arm, either from standing height or higher.
- Nearly half of the fractures are associated with dislocation of the elbow.
- There are three types of fracture:
  1. Type I. Fracture of the coronoid tip; commonly occurs with elbow dislocation and fracture of the radial head, known as the terrible triad.
  2. Type II. Fracture of roughly half of the coronoid process. This is significant because at least half of the coronoid process must be intact for the humeroulnar joint to function.
  3. Type III. Fracture of more than 50% of the coronoid process; nearly always combined with dislocation of the joint.
- You may see fragments of coronoid and must not confuse these with radial head fracture.

Lateral Condyle Fracture

You are briefed by a medical student about a 7-year-old girl who has presented to A&E with a possible fracture of her left arm. The child is clearly in pain and is refusing to move her arm, even with the help of the mother. You gather through your collateral history that she had been running toward her mother for a hug with open arms, when she fell, face down. This description allows you to conclude that her fall was quite possibly on an outstretched arm with her elbow in extension and forearm in abducted position. On examination, the main area of tenderness is the lateral condyle of the humerus. You decide to order an X-ray to investigate.

Typical Findings
- This type of fracture is quite common in children under the age of 10, accounting for roughly 20% of all fractures of the elbow joint.
- Lateral condyle fractures are unstable due to the force that the extensor muscles of the forearm exert on the bone; you may find that even after stabilisation of the joint, some degree of displacement is observed.
- Elbow dislocations in conjunction with this fracture are not uncommon.
- A complication of lateral condyle fracture is non-union. This is due to the nature of the fracture, being intra-articular and immersed in synovial fluid.

Fractures of the Humerus

Proximal Fractures

You are called to A&E to see a 34-year-old man who has been involved in a road traffic accident. He has a GCS of 15 on arrival and is able to give you a detailed history of the incident. You observe that his injuries are relatively minor and although in a lot of pain from his left shoulder, he is otherwise stable and able to communicate. The full physical examination reveals a few cuts and bruises, tender left arm and leg with exacerbation of pain on movement of the left shoulder. Neurological and other examinations prove unremarkable. You request an X-ray of the left shoulder region, which reveals a humeral surgical neck fracture.

Typical Findings
- This is the most common type of fracture of the proximal humerus, which constitutes 5% of all fractures in adults.
- Surgical neck fracture is an extra-capsular fracture, which in contrast to the anatomical neck fracture has adequate blood supply and seldom leads to avascular necrosis.
- Proximal fragment often displays abduction and external rotation due to the action of the muscles attached to the greater tubercle.
- Distal segment appears internally rotated and adducted.

- These types of fractures can be divided into stable and unstable fractures, with the latter occurring due to high-impact blows to the shoulder, displaying involvement of the periosteum and movement between the humeral shaft and fractured head.
- There may be some degree of axillary nerve damage.

Anterior Shoulder Dislocation
A 64-year-old woman is brought to A&E at 2:30 pm, following a fall at home in the early hours of the morning. She appears confused, lethargic and has an obvious abnormal contour of her right shoulder region. After carrying out the initial assessments and addressing her dehydration, you order an X-ray.

Typical Findings
- Most common type of shoulder dislocation.
- Usually seen in the elderly following a fall on an outstretched arm in abducted position.
- Humeral head would be displaced anteriorly and out of the glenohumeral joint; the glenoid will be detached from the labrum.
- AP view on X-ray would show the humeral head positioned under the coracoid process.
- Rotator cuff tear will also be present.
- May or may not be accompanied by the compression fractures of the head/neck or the tuberosities.

Posterior Shoulder Dislocation
You are called to see a patient with profound learning disability who is accompanied by his carer. Through your collateral history, you gather that he is 19 years old and has a history of epilepsy and diabetes. His carer explains that she saw him have "one of his fits" at lunch time and after the episode had ceased, he was complaining of pain in his left shoulder. You decide to examine him fully and request an X-ray to confirm your suspicions of a possible shoulder dislocation.

Typical Findings
- This is a rare type of dislocation and occurs when the arm is in adducted position and internally rotated.
- The internal rotator muscles are much more powerful than the external rotators and a sudden and severe contraction of these muscles can cause the head of the humerus to dislocate.

- Seizure and electrocution are the most common causes.
- It is difficult to pick up signs of this dislocation on physical examination; the head of the humerus can sometimes but not often be palpable under the acromion and the arm cannot usually be externally rotated.
- The axillary view on X-ray would show the humeral head displaced posteriorly to the glenoid fossa and this may appear normal on AP view.

Humeral Shaft Fracture: Holstein–Lewis Fracture
A 40-year-old man is brought to A&E with an injury to his right arm following a football match fight and his attempts to defend his team's poor performance. He appears agitated and distressed and visibly in a lot of pain. On inspection, his arm is very clearly deformed with a large amount of inflammation that he tells you "is getting worse by the minute." He also tells you that he is unable to move his arm in any direction and seems very worried about the "blackening" of his arm below the fracture region. You reassure him that this is an expected case of subcutaneous ecchymosis and after the panic-stricken look he gives you, you explain that it is simply blood accumulating under his skin. You carry out a full examination of the arm, including the skin and neurological function; you detect radial nerve damage in both sensory and motor components and request an X-ray.

Typical Findings
- This is a spiral fracture of the distal 1/3 of the humerus, with the distal fragment displaced anteriorly.
- The radial nerve can be trapped between the fragments of the fracture causing weakness or paralysis: radial nerve palsy.
- Closed reductions are often avoided due to the vulnerability of the radial nerve at the site of the fracture.
- Open reductions are often advised with location, dissection and lateral displacement of the nerve followed by reduction of the fracture and its stabilisation with screws.
- Expected recovery time is 3–4 month.

Key Points

BrachioRadialis: The law of **B-R**
- Function: **B**eer-**R**aising muscle-flexes elbow
- Innervation: **B**reaks the **R**ules of innervations—it is a flexor muscle **B**ut **R**adial (the common nerve innervating the extensor compartment)
- Important relation: **B**ehind the **R**adial nerve in the cubital fossa
- Attachment: **B**ottom of the **R**adius

Flexor digitorum insertion rhyme:
- Superficilias splits in two — to permit profundus passing through!

Median nerve: The muscles of the hand that it innervates: LOAF
- **L**umbricals 1 & 2
- **O**pponens pollicis
- **A**bductor pollicis brevis
- **F**lexor pollicis brevis

Intrinsic muscles of the hand (palmar): **A**ll **F**or **O**ne **A**nd **O**ne **F**or **A**ll
- Thenar:
  Abductor pollicis brevis
  Flexor pollicis brevis
  Opponens pollicis
  Adductor pollicis
- Hypothenar:
  Opponens digiti minimi
  Flexor digiti minimi
  Abductor digiti minimi

Carpal bones of the hand: **S**ome **L**ove **T**o **P**iece **T**ogether, **T**he **C**up **H**older
- **S**caphoid
- **L**unate
- **T**riquetrum
- **P**isiform
- **T**rapezium
- **T**rapezoid
- **C**apitate
- **H**amate

Carpal bones of the hand: Common fracture versus dislocation
- Sca**F**oid: Commonly **F**ractured (leading to avascular necrosis of the proximal part of the bone)
- **L**unate: Commonly dis**L**ocated (leading to median nerve damage)

Interosseous actions: **PAD** & **DAB**
- PAD = **P**almar **AD**duction.
- DAB = **D**orsal **AB**duction

The forearm
- **Common flexor origin**—Medial epicondyle of the humerus
- **Common extensor origin**—Lateral epicondyle of the humerus

Humeral attachment of Latissimus dorsi: **Lady** between two **Majors**
- **Lady:** Latissimus dorsi
- **Majors**: Pectoralis major & teres major

Cubital fossa contents: **M**y **B**ottom's **T**urned **R**ed (Medial → lateral)
- **M**edian nerve
- **B**rachial artery
- **T**endon of biceps
- **R**adial nerve

3 Lower limb

Shalina Mitchell and Somayyeh Shahsavari

> **OBJECTIVES**
> - Bones of the Lower Limb
> - Muscles of the Lower Limb: Attachment, Action and Innervation
> - Joints of the Lower Limb
> - Ligaments of the Lower Limb
> - Clinical Scenarios
> - Key Pointers

The lower limb, unlike the upper, is designed to have a key role in providing structural stability along with the vertebral column. It supports the body weight while limiting the energy expended by the lower limb muscles. The bones here are arranged in a fashion which allows the transfer of body weight between the joints. Locomotion and balance are also major functions for which we depend almost entirely on this part of the body. The bones, joints and muscles within the lower limb must work in concert to allow us stability when standing as well as carrying out the smooth movements of which we are capable. Due to their role in weight-bearing and movement, the bones, joints and muscles of the lower limb are vulnerable to injury. Such injury will have various effects on mobility and independence, particularly in later life.

Table 1 Bones of the Pelvis

Bone	Structure	Muscle attachments	Important features
Pelvis	Acetabulum	–	Formed by fusion of ischium, ilium and pubis; surrounded by acetabular labrum Articulates with head of femur to form hip joint
Ilium	Anterior inferior iliac spine	Rectus femoris (straight head)	Fan-shaped superior portion of pelvis; largest part of hip bone Reflected head of rectus femoris attaches to ilium just superior to acetabulum Inferior to ASIS
	Anterior superior iliac spine (ASIS)	Tensor fasciae latae; iliacus; sartorius	Sits at anterior end of iliac spine
	Gluteal lines: posterior, middle and inferior	–	Lie on outer surface of ilium; form boundaries for areas to which gluteus medius and minimus attach
	Iliac crest	Internal oblique; transversus abdominus; iliocostalis; gluteus maximus; tensor fasciae latae; iliacus; quadratus lumborum; external oblique	"Rim" of ilium; sits at level of L4 vertebra
Ischium	Ischial body	–	Ischium forms posteroinferior portion of hip bone Forms posterior part of acetabulum
	Ischial ramus	Adductor magnus; ischiocavernosus	Inferior boundary of obturator foramen
	Ischial spine	Gemellus superior; coccygeus; levator ani	Projects posteriorly close to junction of ischial ramus and body
	Ischial tuberosity	Gemellus inferior; quadratus femoris; adductor magnus; long head of biceps femoris; semimembranosus; semitendinosus; ischiocavernosus; superficial transverse perineal muscle	Protrudes posteroinferiorly from the body of the ischium
	Obturator foramen and canal	Obturator externus and internus obturator (membrane)	Forms connection between pelvis and adductor canal; allows passage of obturator vessels and nerve out of the pelvis
Pubis	Inferior pubic ramus	Adductor brevis; obturator internus	Extends from inferior part of pubic symphysis; inferior boundary of obturator foramen (with ischium) Unites with ischial ramus to form ischiopubic ramus
	Ischiopubic ramus	Gracilis; adductor part of adductor magnus; compressor urethrae (in women); obturator internus	Rami from both sides form the pubic arch and meet at pubic symphysis; the angle inferior to this point is called the subpubic angle
	Pecten pubis	Pectineus; psoas minor	Ridge on superior pubic ramus
	Pubic body	Pyramidalis; gracilis; adductor brevis and longus; levator ani; external urethral sphincter; pyramidalis	Articulates at the pubic symphysis
	Pubic crest and tubercle	Rectus abdominis (+ pubic symphysis); external oblique; internal oblique; transversus abdominis	Crest—ridge on superior border of body Tubercle—swelling at lateral end of pubic crest
	Superior pubic ramus	–	Extends from pubic body; superior boundary of obturator foramen
Sacrum		Iliocostalis; piriformis; gluteus maximus; iliacus; latissimus dorsi; coccygeus	Formed of five fused bones; connects the hip bones posteriorly; provides stability and strength to pelvis
Coccyx		Gluteus maximus; coccygeus; levator ani	Usually formed of four fused bones; most inferior part of vertebral column

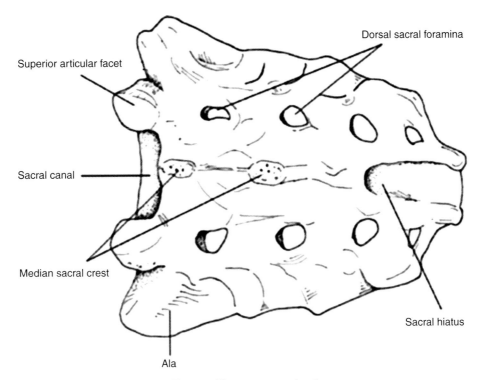

Figure 1a The sacrum; posterior view.

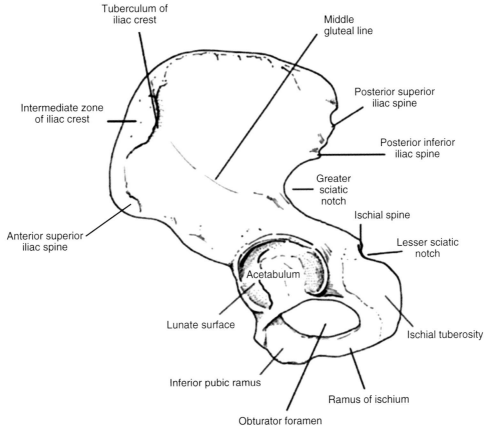

Figure 1b The hip bone.

Table 2 Bones of Lower Limb

Bone	Structure	Muscle attachments	Important features
Femur		–	Femur forms part of both hip and knee joints
	Fovea capitis femoris		Shallow depression in head of femur for ligament of head of femur
	Gluteal tuberosity	Vastus lateralis; gluteus maximus	Lies at superior end of linea aspera
	Greater trochanter	Vastus lateralis; piriformis; obturator internus; gemellus superior and gemellus inferior; gluteus minimus; gluteus medius	Lies at junction of neck and shaft of femur
	Head of femur	–	Has its own arterial supply and ligament Articulates with acetabulum
	Intercondylar fossa	–	Deep notch on posterior surface of femur; location of crossing of cruciate ligaments
	Intertrochanteric crest	Quadratus femoris (quadrate tubercle of intertrochanteric crest)	Connects greater and lesser trochanters on posterior surface of femur
	Intertrochanteric line	Vastus medialis; vastus lateralis	Connects greater and lesser trochanters on anterior surface of femur; attachment site of joint capsule
	Lateral condyle	Lateral head of gastrocnemius; popliteus	Inferior end of femur on lateral side Articulates with lateral condyle of tibia
	Lateral epicondyle	–	Lateral side of femur superior to lateral condyle
	Lateral supracondylar line	Plantaris	Extends from distal end of linea aspera to lateral condyle
	Lesser trochanter	Psoas major; iliacus (iliopsoas)	Conical elevation with rounded tip; distal to neck on posteromedial surface of femur
	Linea aspera	Vastus medialis; vastus lateralis; short head of biceps femoris; adductor longus and brevis; adductor magnus	Double-edged ridge on posterior surface of femur
	Medial condyle	Medial head of gastrocnemius	Inferior end of femur on medial side Articulates with medial condyle of tibia
	Adductor tubercle	Hamstring part of adductor magnus	Medial side of femur superior to medial condyle
	Medial supracondylar line	Vastus medialis; adductor magnus	Ascends from medial epicondyle to medial lip of linea aspera
	Neck of femur	–	Blood vessels supplying femoral head course along neck; vessels vulnerable to damage in femoral neck fracture
	Shaft	Vastus intermedius	–
	Spiral line	Vastus medialis; pectineus; adductor brevis	Extends from lesser trochanter on posterior surface of femur to form medial lip of linea aspera
Fibula	Shaft	Peroneus longus and brevis; extensor hallucis longus; extensor digitorum longus; peroneus tertius; soleus; flexor hallucis longus; tibialis posterior	Fibula is a non-weight-bearing bone
	Head	Peroneus longus; biceps femoris	Proximal end Articulates with tibia
	Lateral malleolus	–	Projection on lateral side of distal fibula; lateral side of ankle joint Articulates with talus
Patella		Vastus medialis; vastus intermedius; vastus lateralis	Sesamoid bone in quadriceps femoris tendon; forms the knee cap
Tibia	Medial condyle	Semimembranosus	Larger, weight-bearing medial bone of leg; smaller at distal end than proximally Articulates with knee, ankle, fibula Prominence on medial side of proximal tibia Articulates with femur (medial condyle)

(Continued)

Table 2 (*Continued*) Bones of Lower Limb

Bone	Structure	Muscle attachments	Important features
	Medial malleolus	–	Projection on medial side of distal tibia; medial side of ankle joint
			Articulates with talus (medial side)
	Lateral condyle	Tibialis anterior; extensor digitorum longus; occasional origin of peroneus longus	Prominence on lateral side of proximal tibia
	Shaft	Flexor digitorum longus; gracilis; soleus; tibialis posterior; sartorius; semitendinosus; popliteus	Articulates with femur (lateral condyle), head of fibula
			–
	Tibial tuberosity	–	Site of insertion of patella tendon

Each lower limb consists of 30 bones. The thigh consists of 1 bone, the leg of 3 bones and the foot of 26, made up of 7 tarsal bones, 5 metatarsals and 14 phalanges. The pelvis consists of the three fused bones of each hip plus the sacrum and coccyx (which may also be classed as part of the vertebral column). The significant features and muscle attachments of these bones are detailed in the tables below and the anatomical arrangement illustrated in the images and sketches below.

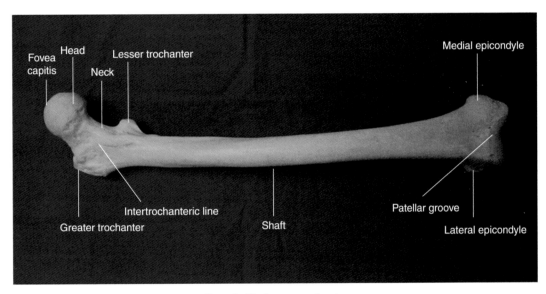

Figure 2a The femur; anterior view.

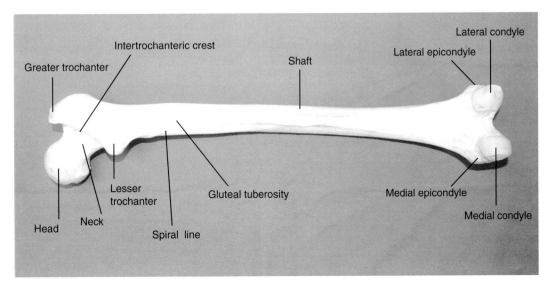

Figure 2b The femur; posterior view.

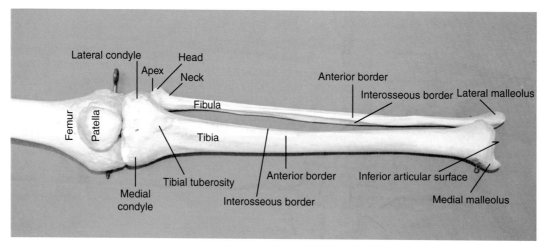

Figure 3a Tibia/fibula and patella; anterior view.

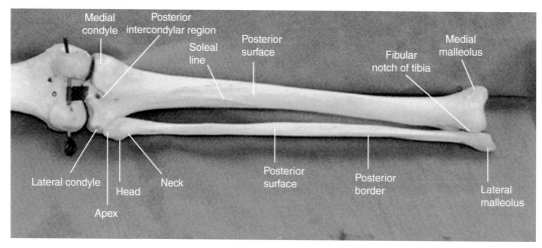

Figure 3b Tibia/fibula and patella; posterior view.

Table 3 Bones of the Foot

Bone	Muscle attachments	Important features
Talus	–	Described as snail-shaped when viewed medially or laterally; size expands posteriorly from domed head Articulates with lateral and medial malleoli
Calcaneus	Abductor hallucis; flexor digitorum brevis; extensor digitorum brevis; abductor digiti minimi; quadratus plantae; gastrocnemius; soleus; plantaris	Supports talus; irregular, box-shaped; calcaneal (Achilles) tendon attached to middle part of bone Articulates with talus, cuboid
Navicular	Tibialis posterior	Contains a medial, rounded tuberosity allowing attachment of tibialis posterior tendon on plantar surface of bone Articulates with cuneiforms, talus

(*Continued*)

Table 3 (Continued) Bones of the Foot

Bone	Muscle attachments	Important features
Cuboid	Flexor hallucis brevis (plantar surface); tibialis posterior	A groove on the plantar surface contains the fibularis longus tendon Articulates with calcaneus, lateral cuneiform, 4th and 5th metatarsals
Medial cuneiform	Tibialis anterior; peroneus longus; tibialis posterior	Articulates with intermediate cuneiform, navicular, 1st metatarsal
Lateral cuneiform	Flexor hallucis brevis	Articulates with intermediate cuneiform, navicular, 3rd metatarsal
Intermediate cuneiform	–	Articulates with lateral and medial cuneiforms, navicular, 2nd metatarsal
Metatarsals	Base of metatarsal 5—flexor digiti minimi brevis Sides and bases of 3 to 5—plantar interossei Bases of 2 to 5—adductor hallucis Sides of 1 to 5—dorsal interossei Base of metatarsal 5—peroneus tertius; peroneus brevis Base of metatarsal 1—peroneus longus, tibialis anterior Bases of 2 to 4—tibialis posterior	Articulate with cuboid, cuneiforms
Phalanges	Great toe • distal phalanx—extensor hallucis longus; flexor hallucis longus • proximal phalanx—extensor digitorum brevis, abductor hallucis, adductor hallucis, flexor hallucis brevis Lateral 4 toes (distal phalanges)—flexor digitorum longus; extensor digitorum longus; middle phalanges—flexor digitorum brevis, proximal phalanges—dorsal interossei; plantar interossei Little toe (proximal phalanx—abductor digiti minimi; flexor digiti minimi brevis	Articulates with metatarsals

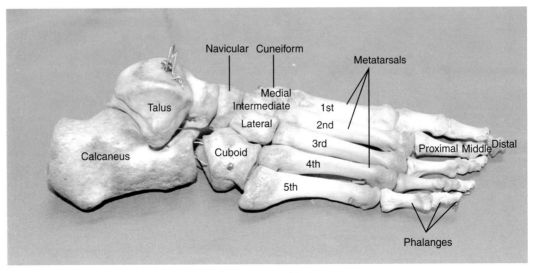

Figure 4a Bones of the foot.

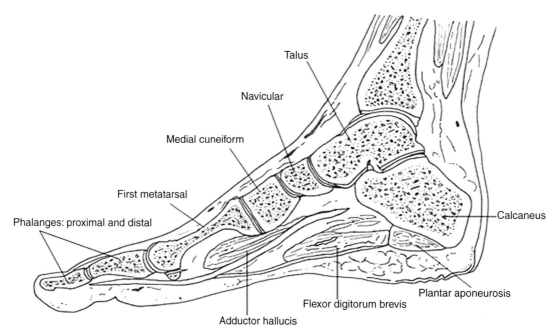

Figure 4b Medial section of foot and ankle.

The muscles of the lower limb are crucial in enabling its complex locomotive function. Various muscles have different roles within the stages of the gait cycle. The muscles are divided into compartments within the thigh and leg. In the thigh, there are medial, anterior and posterior compartments, which are involved in adduction (medial compartment) and flexion and extension (anterior and posterior compartments).

The leg consists of lateral, anterior and posterior compartments, involved in foot eversion, ankle dorsiflexion and toe extension and ankle plantarflexion and toe flexion, respectively. The actions of each muscle, along with its attachments and innervations, are detailed in the tables below. The anatomical arrangements are illustrated in the images and sketches below.

Table 4 Muscles of the Gluteal Region

Muscle	Proximal attachment	Distal attachment	Action	Innervation
Gemellus inferior	Ischial tuberosity	Medial side of greater trochanter of femur with obturator internus tendon (inferior surface)	Lateral rotation of the extended femur. Abduction of flexed femur	Nerve to quadratus femoris (L5, S1)
Gemellus superior	Dorsal surface of ischial spine	Medial side of greater trochanter of femur with obturator internus tendon (superior surface)	Lateral rotation of the extended femur. Abduction of flexed femur	Nerve to obturator internus (L5, S1)
Gluteus maximus	External surface of ilium posterior to posterior gluteal line, posterior iliac crest, dorsal surface of sacrum, lateral margin of coccyx, fascia covering gluteus medius, sacrotuberous ligament	Iliotibial tract of fascia lata and gluteal tuberosity of femur	Extension of flexed femur Stabilisation of femur. Lateral rotation and abduction of thigh	Inferior gluteal nerve (L5, S1, S2)

(Continued)

Table 4 (*Continued*) Muscles of the Gluteal Region

Muscle	Proximal attachment	Distal attachment	Action	Innervation
Gluteus medius	External surface of ilium between anterior and posterior lines	Lateral surface of the greater trochanter of femur	Abduction of femur. Medial rotation of thigh	Superior gluteal nerve (L4, L5, S1)
Gluteus minimus	External surface of ilium between anterior and inferior gluteal lines	Anterolateral aspect of the greater trochanter of femur	Abduction of femur. Medial rotation of thigh	Superior gluteal nerve (L4, L5, S1)
Obturator internus	Internal surface of obturator membrane and surrounding bone	Medial side of greater trochanter of femur	Lateral rotation of the extended femur. Abduction of flexed femur	Nerve to obturator internus (L5, S1)
Piriformis	Anterior surface of the sacrum and sacrotuberous ligament	Superior border of greater trochanter of femur	Lateral rotation of the extended femur. Abduction of flexed femur	Branches from anterior rami of S1, S2, (sometimes L5)
Quadratus femoris	Lateral border of ischial tuberosity	Quadrate tubercle on intertrochanteric crest of the femur	Lateral rotation of femur at hip joint	Nerve to quadratus femoris (L5, S1)
Tensor fasciae latae	Anterior iliac crest, anterior superior iliac spine	Iliotibial tract	Medial rotation and abduction of femur. Stabilisation of knee in extension	Superior gluteal nerve (L4, L5, S1)

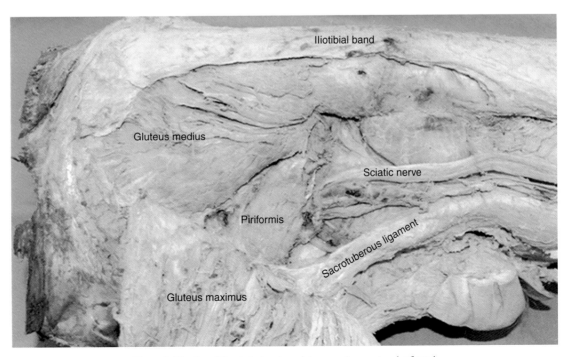

Figure 5 Muscles of the gluteal region; gluteus maximus cut and reflected.

Table 5 Muscles of the Thigh

Muscle	Proximal attachment	Distal attachment	Action	Innervation
Anterior compartment				
Iliacus	Iliac fossa, iliac crest, ala of sacrum, anterior sacroiliac ligaments	Lesser trochanter of femur with psoas major tendon (iliopsoas)	Flexion of femur	Femoral nerve (L2, L3)
Psoas major	Transverse processes of lumbar vertebrae, lateral aspects and intervertebral discs of T12–L5 vertebrae	Lesser trochanter of femur	Flexion of femur Extension of lumbar vertebral column to maintain posture	Anterior rami of L1, L2, L3 nerves
Sartorius	Anterior superior iliac spine	Tibia medial to tibial tuberosity (*pes anserinus*)	Flexion and lateral rotation of femur Flexion of leg at knee joint	Femoral nerve (L2, L3)
Quadriceps				
Rectus femoris	Straight head–anterior inferior iliac spine; reflected head-ilium just superior to the acetabulum	Quadriceps tendon	Flexion of hip and extension of leg at knee joint	Femoral nerve (L2, L3, L4)
Vastus intermedius	Upper two-thirds of anterior and lateral surface of femur	Quadriceps tendon and lateral margin of patella	Extension of leg at knee joint	Femoral nerve (L2, L3, L4)
Vastus lateralis	Intertrochanteric line, greater trochanter, lateral margin of gluteal tuberosity, lateral lip of linea aspera	Quadriceps tendon	Extension of leg at knee joint	Femoral nerve (L2, L3, L4)
Vastus medialis	Intertrochanteric line, spiral line, medial lip of the linea aspera, medial supracondylar line	Quadriceps tendon and medial border of patella	Extension of leg at knee joint	Femoral nerve (L2, L3, L4)
Medial compartment				
Adductor brevis	Body of pubis and inferior pubic ramus	Spiral line and proximal linea aspera	Adduction of femur	Obturator nerve (L2, L3)
Adductor longus	Body of pubis inferior to pubic crest and lateral to pubic symphysis	Middle third of linea aspera of femur	Adduction and medial rotation of femur	Obturator nerve (L2, L3, L4)
Adductor magnus	Adductor part—ischiopubic ramus Hamstring part—ischial tuberosity	Linea aspera, medial supracondylar line Adductor tubercle of femur	Adduction and medial rotation of femur	Obturator nerve (L2, L3, L4) Sciatic nerve (tibial division) (L4)
Gracilis	Body of pubis, ischiopubic ramus	Medial surface of proximal tibia (*pes anserinus*)	Adduction of femur Flexion and medial rotation of leg at knee joint	Obturator nerve (L2, L3)
Obturator externus	External surface of obturator membrane and adjacent bone	Trochanteric fossa of femur	Lateral rotation of femur	Obturator nerve (L3, L4)

(*Continued*)

Table 5 (*Continued*) Muscles of the Thigh

Muscle	Proximal attachment	Distal attachment	Action	Innervation
Pectineus	Pectineal line of pubis (pecten pubis)	Spiral line of femur inferior to lesser trochanter	Adduction and flexion of femur	Femoral nerve (L2, L3); branch of obturator nerve (variable)
Posterior compartment				
Hamstrings				
Biceps femoris	Long head—ischial tuberosity; short head—lateral lip of linea aspera	Head of fibula	Flexion and lateral rotation of leg at knee joint Extension and lateral rotation of femur	Sciatic nerve (L5, S1, S2)
Semimembranosus	Ischial tuberosity	Medial and posterior surface of medial tibial condyle	Flexion of leg at knee joint and extension of femur Medial rotation of (semi)flexed knee	Sciatic nerve (L5, S1, S2)
Semitendinosus	Ischial tuberosity	Medial surface of proximal tibia (*pes anserinus*)	Flexion of leg at knee joint and extension of femur Medial rotation of femur at hip joint and leg at knee joint	Sciatic nerve (L5, S1, S2)

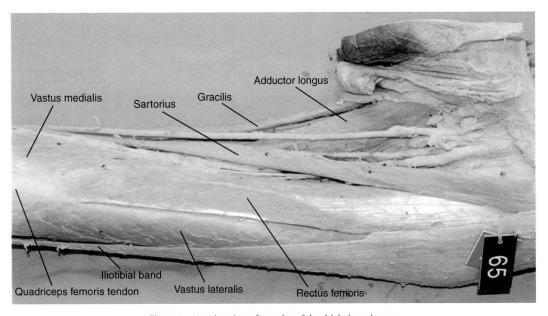

Figure 6a Anterior view of muscles of the thigh: lateral aspect.

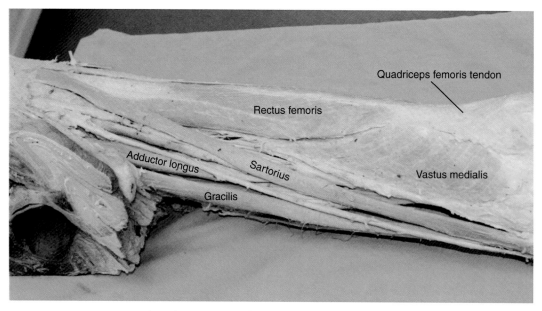

Figure 6b Anterior view of muscles of the thigh: medial aspect.

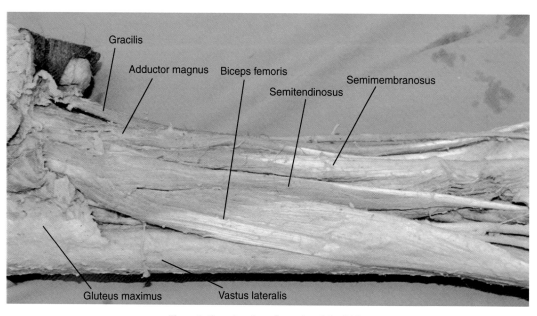

Figure 6c Posterior view of muscles of the thigh.

Table 6 Muscles of the Leg

Muscle	Proximal attachment	Distal Attachment	Action	Innervation
Anterior compartment				
Extensor digitorum longus	Medial surface of fibula, lateral tibial condyle and interosseous membrane	Bases of middle and distal phalanges of lateral four toes	Extension of lateral four toes Dorsiflexion of foot	Deep peroneal (fibular) nerve (L5, S1)
Extensor hallucis longus	Medial surface of fibula and interosseous membrane	Dorsal surface of base of distal phalanx of great toe (hallux)	Extension of great toe Dorsiflexion of foot	Deep peroneal (fibular) nerve (L5, S1)
Peroneus (fibularis) tertius	Medial surface of distal fibula	Dorsomedial surface of base and shaft of 5th metatarsal	Dorsiflexion and eversion of foot	Deep peroneal (fibular) nerve (L5, S1)
Tibialis anterior	Lateral surface and lateral condyle of tibia and interosseous membrane	Medial and plantar surfaces of medial cuneiform and base of 1st metatarsal	Dorsiflexion of foot at ankle joint Inversion of foot	Deep peroneal (fibular) nerve (L4, L5)

(Continued)

Table 6 (*Continued*) Muscles of the Leg

Muscle	Proximal attachment	Distal Attachment	Action	Innervation
Lateral compartment				
Peroneus (fibularis) brevis	Lower two-thirds of lateral surface of fibula	Base of 5th metatarsal	Eversion Dorsiflexion of foot	Superficial peroneal (fibular) nerve (L5, S1, S2)
Peroneus (fibularis) longus	Upper two-thirds of lateral surface and head of fibula	Medial cuneiform and base of 1st metatarsal	Eversion and dorsiflexion of foot	
Posterior compartment				
Gastrocnemius	Lateral head—lateral femoral condyle Medial head—distal femur just superior to medial condyle	Posterior surface of calcaneus via calcaneal tendon	Plantarflexion of foot Flexion of knee	Tibial nerve (S1, S2)
Plantaris	Inferior part of lateral supracondylar line of femur and oblique popliteal ligament of knee	Posterior surface of calcaneus via calcaneal tendon	Weak plantarflexion of foot Flexion of knee	Tibial nerve (S1, S2)
Soleus	Posterior surface of superior third of fibula; soleal line on posterior surface of tibia	Posterior surface of calcaneus via calcaneal tendon	Plantarflexion of foot	Tibial nerve (S1, S2)
Deep compartment				
Flexor digitorum longus	Medial part of posterior surface of tibial shaft	Bases of distal phalanges of the lateral four toes	Flexion of lateral four toes	Tibial nerve (S2, S3)
Flexor hallucis longus	Posterior surface of fibula and inferior portion of interosseous membrane	Base of distal phalanx of great toe (hallux)	Flexion of great toe	
Popliteus	Lateral surface of lateral femoral condyle, lateral meniscus	Posterior surface of tibia above soleal line	Unlocks knee joint (laterally rotates femur on fixed tibia) on commencement of flexion	Tibial nerve (L4, L5, S1)
Tibialis posterior	Posterior surfaces of interosseous membrane and adjacent surfaces of tibia and fibula	Mainly to tuberosity of navicular and adjacent region of medial cunei-form, also to cuboid and bases of 2nd to 4th metatarsals	Inversion and plantarflexion of foot	Tibial nerve (L4, L5)

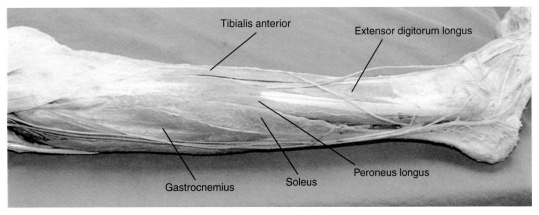

Figure 7a Lateral view of muscles of the leg.

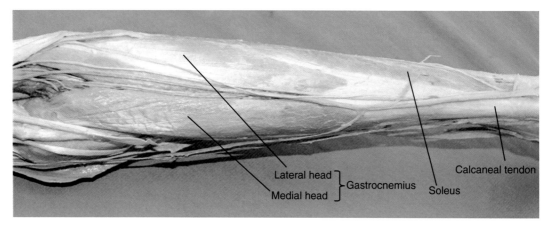

Figure 7b Posterior view of muscles of the leg.

Table 7 Muscles of the Foot

Muscle	Proximal attachment	Distal attachment	Action	Innervation
Dorsal aspect				
Extensor digitorum brevis	Dorsolateral surface of the calcaneus	Base of proximal phalanx of great toe and lateral border of the tendons of extensor digitorum longus of 2nd to 4th toes	Extension of metatarsophalangeal (MTP) joint of great toe Extension of 2nd to 4th toes	Deep fibular nerve (S1, S2)
First layer of sole of foot				
Abductor digiti minimi	Lateral and medial tubercles of calcaneal tuberosity and plantar aponeurosis	Lateral side of base of proximal phalanx of little toe	Abduction and flexion of little toe at MTP joint	Lateral plantar nerve (S1, S2, S3)
Abductor hallucis	Medial process of calcaneal tuberosity, flexor retinaculum and plantar aponeurosis	Medial side of base of proximal phalanx of great toe	Abduction and flexion of great toe at MTP joint	Medial plantar nerve (S1, S2, S3)
Flexor digitorum brevis	Medial aspect of calcaneal tuberosity and plantar aponeurosis	Middle phalanges of lateral four toes	Flexion of lateral four toes at proximal interphalangeal joint	Medial plantar nerve (S1, S2, S3)
Second layer of sole of foot				
Lumbricals	First lumbrical—medial side of flexor digitorum longus tendon; second, third and fourth lumbricals—adjacent sides of flexor digitorum longus tendons	Medial aspect of extensor hoods of 2nd to 5th toes	Flexion of MTP joint Extension of interphalangeal joints	First lumbrical – medial plantar nerve; second, third and fourth lumbricals – lateral plantar nerve (S2, S3)
Quadratus plantae	Medial surface of calcaneus and lateral process of calcaneal tuberosity	Lateral side of flexor digitorum longus tendon	Assists flexor digitorum longus tendon in flexion of 2nd to 4th toes	Lateral plantar nerve (S1, S2, S3)

(Continued)

Table 7 (*Continued*) Muscles of the Foot

Muscle	Proximal attachment	Distal attachment	Action	Innervation
Third layer of sole of foot				
Adductor hallucis	Transverse head— plantar ligaments of metatarsophalangeal joints of lateral three toes; oblique head— bases of metatarsals of 2nd to 5th toes	Lateral side of base of proximal phalanx of great toe	Adduction of great toe at MTP joint	Lateral plantar nerve (S2, S3)
Flexor digiti minimi brevis	Base of 5th metatarsal	Lateral side of base of proximal phalanx of little toe	Flexion of little toe at MTP joint	Lateral plantar nerve (S2, S3)
Flexor hallucis brevis	Plantar surface of cuboid and lateral cuneiform	Lateral and medial sides of base of proximal phalanx of the great toe	Flexion of MTP joint of the great toe	Medial plantar nerve (S1, S2)
Fourth layer of sole of foot				
Dorsal interossei	Sides of adjacent metatarsals 1–5	Bases of proximal phalanges of 2nd to 4th toes	Abduction of 2nd to 4th toes at MTP joints Flexion of MTP joints	Lateral plantar nerve; first and second dorsal interossei also innervated by deep peroneal (fibular) nerve (S2, S3)
Plantar interossei	Medial sides and bases of metatarsals 3–5	Bases of proximal phalanges of 3rd to 5th toes	Adduction of 3rd to 5th toes at the MTP joints Flexion of MTP joints	Lateral plantar nerve (S2, S3)

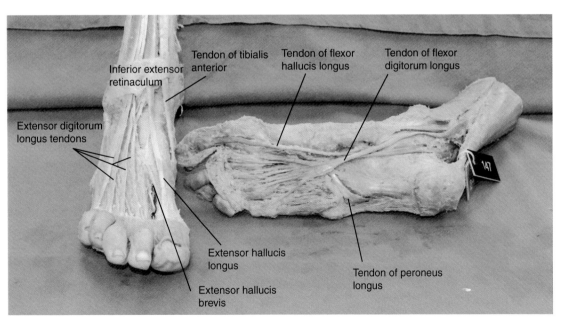

Figure 8 Dorsal and plantar views of the tendons of foot muscles.

The crucial role of the lower limbs in movement and weight-bearing means that the joints of this region are susceptible to wear-and-tear with age. The effects of these changes will vary with individuals but can be considerably disabling. The lower limb contains three large joints, namely hip, knee and ankle and a number of smaller joints within the foot. The type and articulations of each joint, along with its action and important features, are detailed in the tables below.

Table 8 Joints of the Lower Limb

Joint	Type	Articulations	Action	Important features
Ankle	Synovial hinge	Talus Lateral malleolus of fibula Medial malleolus of tibia	Dorsiflexion Plantarflexion	Most stable when foot is dorsiflexed Blood supply: posterior tibial artery, dorsalis pedis
Calcaneocuboid	Synovial plane	Distal surface of calcaneus Proximal surface of cuboid	Inversion of foot Eversion of foot Circumduction	
Cuneonavicular	Synovial plane	Distal navicular surface Bases of cuneiforms	Little movement permitted	
Hip	Synovial ball-and-socket	Head of femur Acetabulum of hip bone	Flexion Extension Abduction Adduction Rotation	Reinforced by capsular ligaments Blood supply: Cruciate anastomosis—inferior gluteal artery, medial and lateral circumflex femoral arteries, ascending perforator from profunda femoris artery; also branch of obturator artery to head of femur (atrophies with age)
Interphalangeal	Synovial hinge	Proximal interphalangeal (PIP) joints: formed by articulations between proximal and middle phalanges Distal interphalangeal (DIP) joints: formed by articulations between middle and distal phalanges	Flexion Extension	
Knee	Synovial hinge	Femur Tibia Patella	Flexion Extension Slight medial and lateral rotation when flexed	Has two articulations—one between femur and tibia and the other between femur and patella Blood supply: Femoral and popliteal arteries; superior medial , superior lateral, inferior medial, inferior lateral and descending genicular arteries, recurrent branch of anterior tibial artery
Metatarsophalangeal (MTP)	Synovial condyloid joint	Head of metatarsal Base of proximal phalanx	Flexion of toes Extension of toes Abduction of toes Adduction of toes	
Subtalar (or talocalcaneal)	Synovial plane	Inferior surface of body of talus Superior surface of calcaneus	Inversion of foot Eversion of foot	
Talocalcaneonavicular	Synovial	Head of talus Calcaneus Navicular	Gliding movements Rotatory movements	Talonavicular portion of joint is ball-and-socket type

(Continued)

Table 8 (*Continued*) Joints of the Lower Limb

Joint	Type	Articulations	Action	Important features
Tarsometatarsal	Synovial plane	Distal tarsal bones Proximal ends of metatarsal bones	Movement limited to gliding of bones against each other	
Sacroiliac	Compound joint—anterior synovial joint and posterior syndesmosis	Sacrum Ilium	Only limited mobility allowed at joint (slight gliding and rotary movements)	Strong and weight-bearing

The ligaments of the lower limb are particularly vulnerable to damage during sports and exercise. Some of the more common injuries are covered in the Clinical Scenarios section. The attachments and functions of each ligament are detailed in the tables below.

Table 9 Ligaments of Lower Limb

Ligament	Attachments	Function
Hip joint		
Acetabular labrum	Fibrocartilage rim—attached to margin of acetabulum	Increases depth of acetabulum
Iliofemoral (Y-shaped)	Anterior inferior iliac spine and margin of acetabulum Intertrocanteric line of femur	Prevents hyperextension of femur at hip during standing, limits lateral rotation, reinforces and strengthens the joint (strongest ligament in the body)
Ischiofemoral	From ischial wall of acetabulum Neck of femur	Slackens during abduction, tenses during adduction, strengthens articular capsule Limits extension of hip joint, limits medial rotation
Ligament of head of femur (ligamentum teres) (flat, triangular band)	Acetabular notch and transverse acetabular ligament Fovea capitis of femur	Usually contains small artery to head of femur (from obturator artery), limits adduction, not significant in strengthening hip joint
Pubofemoral	Pubic part of acetabulum rim Neck of femur	Prevents over-abduction of femur at hip joint, strengthens articular capsule Limits lateral rotation, limits extension of joint, tightens during extension and abduction
Transverse ligament of acetabulum	Crosses over acetabular notch, connected with ligament of head of femur and articular capsule	Part of acetabular labrum
Knee		
Extra-capsular		
Arcuate popliteal	Posterior aspect of fibular head Intercondylar area of tibia and lateral epicondyle of femur	Strengthens joint capsule posterolaterally Permits passage of tendon of popliteus
Lateral (fibular) collateral (LCL)	Lateral epicondyle of femur Lateral side of head of fibula	Contributes to stability when standing (taut in full extension), permits and limits rotation at the knee
Oblique popliteal	Posterior to medial tibial condyle Lateral femoral condyle, reflection from insertion of semimembranosus	Reinforces joint capsule posteriorly

(*Continued*)

Table 9 (*Continued*) Ligaments of Lower Limb

Ligament	Attachments	Function
Patellar ligament	Apex of patella Tibial tuberosity	Strengthens anterior surface of joint; insertion of quadriceps femoris muscles
Medial (tibial) collateral (MCL)	Medial epicondyle of femur Medial condyle and superior part of the medial surface of the tibia Also attached to medial meniscus	Contributes to stability when standing (taut in full extension), permits and limits rotation at the knee, weaker than LCL and more susceptible to damage
Intra-articular		
Anterior cruciate	Anterior intercondylar area of tibia Posterior part of medial surface of lateral condyle of femur	Limits knee hyperextension, prevents posterior displacement of the femur on the tibia, limits medial rotation
Posterior cruciate	Posterior intercondylar area of tibia Anterior part of lateral surface of medial condyle of femur	Prevents posterior sliding of tibia and anterior sliding of femur when knee flexed (v. imp when walking down stairs or steep incline), prevents hyperflexion of knee joint, limits medial rotation, stronger of the cruciate ligaments
Transverse ligament	Anterior edge of medial meniscus Anterior edge of lateral meniscus	Tethers menisci to each other during movements of knee
Ankle and foot		
Anterior talofibular	Anterior margin of lateral malleolus Neck of talus	Stabilises ankle joint, prevents anterior displacement of talus in relation to fibula and tibia, resists inversion when foot is plantar flexed
Calcaneofibular	Posteromedial side of lateral malleolus Tubercle on lateral surface of calcaneus	Stabilises subtalar joint and limits inversion
Deep transverse metatarsal	Heads of metatarsal bones	Link heads of metatarsals together, enabling metatarsals to act as a unified structure
Interosseous talocalcaneal	Groove between articular facets of under surface of talus Corresponding depression on upper surface of calcaneus (tarsal canal)	Stabilises subtalar joint, reinforces capsule of talocalcaneonavicular joint posteriorly
Lateral talocalcaneal	Lateral surface of talus Lateral surface of calcaneus	Stabilises subtalar joint
Long plantar	Inferior surface of calcaneus Inferior surface of cuboid Superficial fibres extend to bases of metatarsal bones	Resists depression of lateral arch of foot, supports calcaneocuboid joint
Medial/deltoid	Medial malleolus Adjacent talus, calcaneus and navicular	Stabilises ankle joint during eversion and prevents subluxation of the joint
Medial talocalcaneal	Medial tubercle of back of talus Back of sustentaculum tali	Stabilises subtalar joint
Plantar calcaneocuboid (short plantar)	Calcaneal tubercle Inferior surface of cuboid	Resists depression of lateral arch of foot, supports calcaneocuboid joint
Plantar calcaneonavicular (spring ligament)	Anterior margin of sustentaculum tali Plantar surface of navicular	Supports head of talus, resists depression of medial arch of foot, reinforces capsule of talocalcaneonavicular joint inferiorly
Posterior talocalcaneal	Lateral tubercle of talus Upper and medial part of calcaneus	Stabilises subtalar joint
Posterior talofibular	Medial side of lateral malleolus Posterior process of the talus	Stabilises ankle joint, prevents posterior and rotatory subluxation of the talus
Talonavicular	Neck of talus Dorsal surface of navicular bone	Reinforces capsule of talocalcaneonavicular joint superiorly

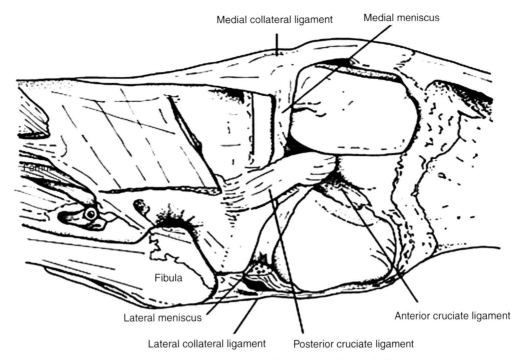

Figure 9a Sketch of the posterior view of the knee joint; showing the ligaments.

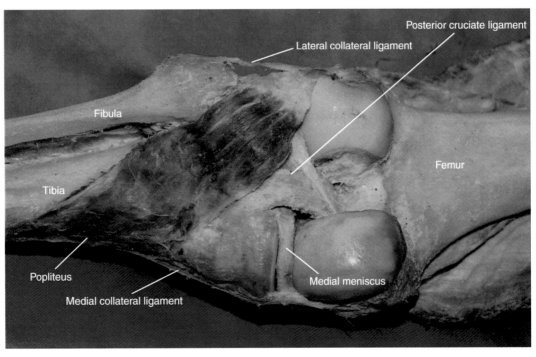

Figure 9b Posterior knee joint.

CLINICAL SCENARIOS

Ankle Injuries

Weber Type A Fracture

Mr J, a 28-year-old builder, was playing football for his local team when he fell, injuring himself. He was brought to A&E by ambulance with a closed fracture of his right ankle. He appears to be in a lot of pain, particularly on palpation and tells you that he is unable to put any "pressure" on his foot. Apart from minor bruises, he has not sustained any other injuries, there is no evidence of neurological compromise and both the dorsalis pedis and posterior tibial pulse are present. His X-ray shows a type A Weber fracture.

Typical Findings

The Weber classification is a system based on lateral malleolar fractures, of which there are three types:

- Type A
  ○ Fracture is below ankle joint involving the lateral malleolus.
  ○ No damage to tibiofibular syndesmosis or the deltoid ligament.
  ○ Mostly stable.
- Type B
  ○ Fracture is at the ankle joint level; involves the fibula, medial malleolus and often the deltoid ligament.

○ The tibiofibular syndesmosis may be intact or incompletely compromised.

○ Stability is variable.

- Type C

○ Fracture is above the ankle joint level.

○ Damage to the tibiofibular syndesmosis with widening of the distal tibiofibular region.

○ Definite medial malleolus and deltoid ligament involvement.

○ Unstable.

Plantar Fasciitis

A 22-year-old man comes to your surgery complaining of a pain in his foot. He tells you that he is training for the marathon and is finding it difficult to stick to his usual program for the last couple of weeks, as the pain is getting worse. He describes the pain as being quite sharp at the start of his run and focused on his heel, travelling down the sole of his foot and easing gradually through training. Mostly, however, the pain returns as a deep, dull ache when he stops running, and 3 days ago he noticed the area was "swelling and becoming a bit stiff." On examination, palpation of the medial tubercle of the calcaneus and passive dorsiflexion of the foot is painful.

Typical Findings

- Repetitive stretching motion of the plantar region of the foot is the main cause, as seen in running.
- Can cause pathological symptoms such as inflammation and, if continued, degenerative changes of the plantar tendon.
- Errors in training methods, wrong type of foot wear and intensive training on hard surfaces are all risk factors.

Turf Toe

A 31-year-old man with a black belt in karate comes to your GP surgery complaining of pain and discomfort in his right big toe. He tells you that he was in a mock combat about 2 weeks ago and attempted to kick with his right leg and missed, hitting a wooden pillar behind his opponent. You gather from his explanation that his right MTP joint must have been in hyperextension and valgus position. The pain has stopped him from going to daily karate sessions, despite trying, and he is finding it hard to put weight on his toe when walking.

Typical Findings

- This type of injury causes MT joint capsule torsion that in turn causes subluxation of the first MTP joint.
- The mechanism of injury is most commonly through hyperextension of the first MTP joint but may also result from hyperflexion.

Achilles Tendon Rupture

A 21-year-old female was diagnosed with lupus and started on methyl prednisolone pulse therapy for 3 days, which was then followed by a lower dose of oral prednisolone daily. Her symptoms began to improve and her WCC returned to normal level. Following her discharge from hospital, she began noticing a "cold feeling" on the back of her left leg that was accompanied by severe pain over the heel and this prompted her to return to her GP for a check-up. The physical examination of the left leg revealed a 3-cm posterior gap palpable above the calcaneus, and the dorsalis pedis pulse was absent. Spontaneous Achilles tendon rupture was suspected and confirmed following an MRI.

Typical Findings

- It can happen suddenly resulting from overstretch of the tendon or following chronic inflammation such as tendonitis.
- Weak calf muscles shortening when overused can exert more force on the tendon than it can tolerate, leading to spontaneous rupture.
- Most vulnerable position is the foot in dorsiflexed position with the lower leg moving forwards and calf muscles contracting.
- A "pop" sound may be heard.
- It is suggested that there is a correlation between corticosteroid use and this type of tendon rupture; some studies have shown this association with long-term use only, and others have reported cases following an initial high dose of the drug.

Grade I Ankle Inversion Injury/Sprain

A 20-year-old man has come to your GP clinic following a fall on uneven ground when hiking the day before. He tells you that he was walking uphill and lost his balance as his right foot touched the ground and he fell on his side with his right foot twisted inwards. He has found weight-bearing painful but not impossible and describes the pain as 5/10 and constant, which is controllable with paracetamol. On examination, the right foot looks moderately swollen and the lateral aspect of the ankle joint is tender to palpation; there is no sign of bruising or instability of the joint. You suspect grade I inversion injury and assure your patient that the use of splint or cast is not necessary. You ensure he understands the importance of resting his ankle and not returning to sporting activities for about 2 weeks, icing and elevating the foot and walking as tolerated. You also ask him to come back and see you if any of his symptoms persist longer than 2 weeks.

Typical Findings

- Inversion ankle injuries are very common and are graded according to severity:

○ Grade I. Mild injury; some swelling and pain but weight-bearing is usually possible without great difficulty. High-impact activities will be painful as the ligaments are stretched beyond their normal range. Although microscopic tears may have occurred, ankle stability is not affected.

○ Grade II. Moderate injury; more obvious swelling is seen with some bruising with more intense pain. It may be difficult to elicit movement in the joint; walking may still be possible unaided but severity of pain will be the deciding factor. Partial tearing of ligaments will be involved but stability of the ankle may still be intact.

○ Grade III. Severe injury; there is significant bruising, swelling and extreme pain due to complete ligament tear. The bruising may be visible on other parts of the foot, as blood begins to pool and weight-bearing without assistance will be extremely difficult as ankle joint stability is lost.

- Grades II and III will require splint/cast as well as physical therapy.
- The three ligaments damaged in this type of injury are the anterior talofibular, posterior talofibular and calcaneofibular ligaments. The anterior talofibular is the most commonly damaged ligament in inversion injuries.
- One mnemonic for remembering the immediate treatment of any ankle sprain is PER-ICE:
  - P = *Protected walking* such as cast boots or crutches
  - E = *Elevation* of foot above the level of the heart
  - R = *Rest* from intensive activities and exercise
  - I = *Ice*; this is important within the first couple of days as it can help reduce inflammation
  - C = *Compression;* this also helps with containing inflammation and promoting healing
  - E = *Early mobilisation* prevents the usual stiffness experienced posthealing

Knee Injuries/Fractures

Baker's Cyst
A 52-year-old man presents to A&E with a 4-day history of painful and swollen right calf. He denies shortness of breath, cough and chest pain and has no previous history of his current complaint. He does not have any significant medical problems and is on no medication at the moment.

On examination, the right knee is moderately swollen but the range of movements is intact. There is no evidence of joint effusion or palpable masses. The right calf is tender and erythematous with clear swelling, when compared to the left calf. You suspect DVT and request an ultrasound, which is negative. You then request an arthrogram, which confirms the diagnosis of ruptured Baker's/Popliteal cyst.

Typical Findings
- Baker's cyst most often presents as a painless popliteal mass in the posteromedial knee region, which transilluminates.
- The mass is not a true cyst as it is actually a distention of gastrocnemio-semimembranosus bursa due to accumulation of synovial fluid.
- The mass can become hardened when extending the knee and soft on flexion (Foucher's sign).
- Factors that must be taken into account are
  - Skin changes at the site of the mass. Think haemangioma, dermatofibrosarcoma, etc.
  - If the mass is very large or seems tethered, think malignancy.
- A ruptured Baker's cyst can resemble DVT to a degree that clinical examination would not be able to offer a definite diagnosis. It is vital to rule out DVT prior to any further investigations.
- This type of cyst is common in the elderly and is often seen in those with degenerative diseases such as rheumatoid arthritis. (Inflammation can lead to increased production of synovial fluid.)

Patellofemoral Pain Syndrome/Runner's Knee
Ms P is a 42-year-old woman with a BMI of 27, who presented to her GP with a 2-week history of left knee pain. The pain was on the right anterior side of the knee and worsened on walking downstairs and sitting for a prolonged amount of time. She admitted to taking some simple over-the-counter pain killers but this had not proven significant in controlling her symptoms. There was no history of trauma.

On examination, there was no evidence of inflammation or bruising to the knee joint. The patella was laterally deviated and this was most obvious when Ms P was lying down and when asked to flex her knee. The range of movement of the knee was normal and pain-free. Pain was noted on compression of the patella and the rest of the examination proved unremarkable.

Typical Findings
- The exact mechanism of patellofemoral pain (PFP) is not well understood but the generally accepted explanation is that the manner in which the patella moves along the groove of femur can cause cartilage irritation and hence, pain.
- This is also known as "runner's knee" and that is because repetitive overloading of the knee can result in pressure on the joint.
- Flat or pronating feet also increase stress on the knee joint, resulting in PFP.
- Another underlying cause could be the disproportionate strength in the quadriceps muscle fibres; stronger outer than inner fibres. As well as increasing stress on the knee joint directly, this can cause tightening of the iliotibial band and worsen the problem.
- Q-angle is also a factor. This refers to the angle of the femur and in some people it can be wider than normal leading to a "knock-kneed" manifestation that is known as genu valgum. Individuals with genu valgum will experience higher knee stress on straightening their legs due to the patella being forced laterally.

O'Donoghue's Unhappy Triad
A 20-year-old man is brought to A&E following an injury sustained while playing for his local American an team. He tells you that he was badly "clipped" from the right; he then felt his right knee give way followed by excruciating pain. Examination reveals swelling of the joint, decreased range of movement and instability. You suspect serious injury and order an MRI of the knee; the results show a tear in the anterior cruciate ligament (ACL), the medial collateral ligament (MCL) and the medial meniscus.

Typical Findings
- Tear of the ACL is the most significant of the three injuries as the stability of the knee is lost as a result; it may take up to 9 months post-operation to see any substantial results.
- No muscles are involved in this injury but rehabilitation post-operation may be focused on the quadriceps femoris to help enhance stability and strength in the knee joint.

Genu Varum/Bow Legs
A 76-year-old man comes to your GP clinic complaining of pain on walking and standing and the gradual decrease in his ability to "sit on the floor" comfortably. He tells you that he is planning a trip "back home to India" and is concerned that this

pain may stop him from enjoying his time there. He is particularly concerned about using the "Indian toilets" that require squatting as he is finding this movement particularly difficult. He has a 12-year history of diabetes, a BMI of 32 and a 6-year history of osteoarthritis (OA) and is otherwise fit and well. You examine the patient in lying down position with the legs extended and ankles joined together; inspection alone shows lateral rotation of the knees and patellae facing outwards in both knees. The distance between the two knees in same position is 3.4 cm and the plumb line test shows both medial malleoli to lie medial to this line. You request an X-ray of both lower limbs in order to carry out a more accurate measurement of the degree of deformity in the knees. The results show OA in both knees, particularly the medial condyles.

Typical Findings
- This condition is normal in infancy and it is usually corrected within the first 2 to 3 years of life.
- In children, this is closely associated with rickets.
- In the elderly, this is usually due to OA affecting the medial aspect of the knee joint more than the lateral; this can be progressively worsening.
- Surgical intervention is often the only option in the elderly and total knee replacement may be necessary depending on severity of deformity and its effect on the patient's quality of life.
- Plumb line test—a line is drawn from anterior superior iliac spine to the centre of patella and finally to the medial malleolus. Usually, these three structures are perfectly aligned but in genu varum, the medial malleolus lies medial to this line.

Hip and Thigh Injuries

Femoral Stress Fracture
An 18-year-old man complains of pain in the anterior region of his left thigh. He plays semi-professional football for his local team and says that his symptoms started with a "pulling" sensation following practice before a big game 8 days ago. He denies trauma. On examination, there is evidence of moderate swelling over rectus femoris with pain exacerbated by palpation of the region. There is also pain during active hip flexion and extension but no pain was elicited during internal and external rotation of the hip. The rest of the examination including neurological examination was unremarkable.

You diagnose rectus femoris strain and discharge him without further investigation. You ensure he is advised to rest and use ice-packs for cooling the muscle. He returns in 10-days with no improvements and you repeat the physical examinations with no change in results and hence order an X-ray. The results reveal callus formation in the middle of the left femur, which is consistent with a stress fracture of this region.

Typical Findings
- Stress fracture results from a repetitive, non-traumatic stress placed on a bone.
- The fracture may be partial or complete.
- The exact mechanism underlying this type of fracture is not well understood but it has been suggested that when a muscle is fatigued, its shock-absorbing

quality is lowered, causing an increased load transfer to the bone.
- Some of the risk factors are
  o Sudden increase in training intensity
  o Inappropriate footwear
  o Malnutrition

Slipped Capital Femoral Epiphysis
A 13-year-old boy complains of pain and discomfort in his left hip and knee that has been on-going for about 3 weeks. He says that the pain is exacerbated by jumping or running but that he can walk and put pressure on his left leg despite the pain. He denies any trauma and has no significant past medical history. You measure his height and weight and calculate his BMI to be 31. On examination, the child's gait is slightly altered; the left leg is externally rotated and there is reduced internal rotation of the hip with exaggerated external rotation. The left leg is also shorter than the right and there is some evidence of muscle wasting in the affected leg's thigh muscles.

You order an X-ray of both hips for comparison that shows epiphyseal line widening in the left hip. There is no evidence of pelvic fracture or any other complications in either hip. You also order relevant blood tests to check thyroid function and growth hormone levels.

Typical Findings
- This condition is seen commonly in adolescents (particularly males) and it is characterised by the instability of the growth plate.
- It can present acutely with spontaneous slippage of the growth plate and difficulty in weight-bearing with extreme pain or chronically with gradual slippage and possible weight-bearing on the affected leg.
- It may be unilateral or bilateral and is greatly associated with obesity in children. It usually affects the non-dominant leg first.
- Other risk factors include hypothyroidism, hypopituitarism and growth hormone deficiency.
- You should always have Perthe's disease in mind as a possible differential diagnosis as well as osteomyelitis.
- Knee pain associated with this is referred pain from the hip but a full lower limb examination should always be carried out.
- Chondrolysis and avascular necrosis of the epiphysis are the two serious complications of this condition.
- The higher the degree of slippage, the poorer the prognosis.

Intracapsular Fracture of Neck of Femur
A 76-year-old woman is brought to A&E following a minor fall and the sudden inability to "put any weight on the right leg." She complains of severe pain in the right knee and some pain in the right hip region. She has a history of Parkinson's, dementia, depression and rheumatoid arthritis.

On examination, the right leg appears shorter and is externally rotated and pain in the hip and knee is exacerbated by movement in all directions. You suspect a fracture and order an AP pelvis and lateral hip X-rays. The results reveal a grade II intracapsular fracture.

Typical Findings

- Hip fractures are very common in the elderly, particularly those with a history of osteoporosis, Parkinson's and arthritis as they are more prone to falls.
- In a young person, this type of fracture usually follows a high-impact injury.
- It is common for intracapsular fractures to present clinically as knee pain only or a combination of knee and hip pain.
- There are many ways of classifying these fractures, one of which is the Garden classification as seen on X-ray: Garden I–IV.
    I. Angulated trabeculae seen with no displacement of head of femur
    II. Trabeculae intact but a fracture is seen running from superior to inferior cortex; no displacement of femoral head is observed
    III. Complete fracture line is visible and there is a slight displacement of head of femur; it may be rotated
    IV. Complete femoral head displacement is clearly visible

Key Points

- When administering intramuscular injections in the gluteal region, it is important to avoid the sciatic nerve. The safest area for injection is the upper outer quadrant of the buttock.
- In the anatomical position, the pelvis is positioned at an angle (tilted slightly forwards) so that the anterior superior iliac spine (ASIS) and the pubic symphysis are in the same vertical plane.
- The femoral triangle is located in the medial region of the proximal thigh and contains the femoral nerve, artery and veins. Its borders are inguinal ligament (superiorly), adductor longus (medially) and sartorius (laterally).
- The contents of the tarsal tunnel posterior to the medial malleolus can be remembered using the mnemonic "**T**om, **D**ick **AN**d **H**arry," which stands for (from anterior to posterior) **t**ibialis posterior, flexor **d**igitorum longus, posterior tibial **a**rtery, tibial **n**erve and flexor **h**allucis longus.
- The arrangement of the tarsal bones (superior to inferior and medial to lateral) can be remembered using the following mnemonic: **T**iger **C**ubs **N**eed **MILC** (**T**alus, **c**alcaneus, **n**avicular, **m**edial, **i**ntermediate and **l**ateral cuneiforms, **c**uboid.

4 The core

Shalina Mitchell and Somayyeh Shahsavari

OBJECTIVES
- Bones of the Core
- Muscles of the Core
- Joints of the Core
- Ligaments of the Core
- Clinical Scenarios
- Key Pointers

The core comprises the back, thorax and abdomen. It contains most of the internal organs of the body and as such has a significant protective role. The bones of the back, the vertebral column, house the spinal cord and the proximal portions of the spinal nerves, which provide a neural pathway from the brain to the rest of the body. Damage here can lead to significant pain and morbidity and even paralysis. The vertebral column supports the trunk and shares the roles of supporting the body's weight and maintaining posture, with the lower limbs. The bony composition of the thorax affords a degree of protection to the heart and lungs within it while the organs within the abdomen are encased by layers of muscle. Both of these arrangements afford advantages clinically. The bony landmarks of the thorax are crucial in clinical examination of this area and the lack of bone in the abdomen allows for more effective palpation of the organs there.

Table 1 Bones of the Core

Bone	Structure	Muscle attachments	Important features
Vertebral column			
Vertebra	Intervertebral foramina	–	Created by adjacent superior and inferior vertebral notches Sit between pedicles Allow passage of spinal nerve roots, vessels (arteries and veins) and contain dorsal root ganglia
	Lamina	–	Dorsal part of the wall of the vertebral foramen (forms vertebral arch)
	Pars interarticularis	–	Between the superior and inferior articular processes Site of pars fractures
	Pedicle	–	Part of the wall of the vertebral foramen (forms vertebral arch) Marked by superior and inferior vertebral notches
	Spinous processes	Serratus posterior (inferior and superior); splenius; spinalis (thoracic, cervical); interspinales (cervical, lumbar); trapezius (C7–T12); latissimus dorsi (T7–L5); rhomboid major (T2–T5) and minor (T1); iliocostalis; transversospinalis	Arise in midline from junction of laminae, project dorsally
	Superior and inferior articular processes (zygapophyses)	–	Each have an articular facet Project inferiorly and superiorly from junction between pedicle and lamina Form zygopophyseal joints—superior processes articulate with inferior processes of the vertebra above
	Transverse process	Levatores costarum; quadratus lumborum; longissimus; spinalis (cervical); transversospinalis; intertransversarii (C, L); psoas major; splenius cervicis; iliocostalis (cervical)	Bilateral Extends from junction between pedicle and lamina Thoracic: articulate with ribs to form costovertebral joints
	Vertebral body	Psoas major and minor (lumbar only); diaphragm	Supports body weight, size increases inferiorly to bear increasing body weight Articulate with intervertebral discs superiorly and inferiorly
	Vertebral canal	–	Contains the spinal cord, meninges, fat, spinal nerve roots and blood vessels
	Vertebral notches	–	Inferior and superior indentations formed by the inferior and superior surfaces of the pedicles Become intervertebral foramina between adjacent vertebrae
Lumbar vertebra		Large, thick vertebral body; triangular foramen; long slender transverse processes with accessory processes on bases; articular processes with superior and inferior facets directed posteromedially and anterolaterally, respectively; short spinous process	
Thoracic vertebra		Heart-shaped vertebral body with bilateral demifacets for articulation with rib heads (atypical thoracic vertebrae have only one costal facet), small vertebral canal relative to lumbar and cervical vertebrae, transverse processes with costal facets for articulation with tubercles of ribs (excluding T10–T12) long spinous process angled posteroinferiorly	
Ribs and sternum			
Ribs	Angle	Iliocostalis	–
	Costal groove	Internal and innermost intercostal muscles	Contains intercostal vessels and intercostal nerve
	Head	–	2 facets—one articulates with corresponding vertebra; one articulates with vertebra superior to it
	Neck	–	Sits between head and tubercle

(Continued)

Table 1 (*Continued*) Bones of the Core

Bone	Structure	Muscle attachments	Important features
	Shaft	External oblique; internal oblique; quadratus lumborum (12th); subcostales; levatores costarum; intercostal muscles; pectoralis minor (3rd to 5th); serratus anterior (1st to 8th); serratus posterior (inferior and superior); longissimus; latissimus dorsi (10th to 12th); subclavius (1st)	Has a sharp inferior margin and a smooth, rounded superior region
	Tubercle	–	*Articular part* articulates with transverse process of corresponding vertebra and non-articular part allows attachment of costotransverse ligament 1–7: vertebrosternal (true) ribs—attach to sternum via costal cartilages 8–10: vertebrochondral (false) ribs—costal cartilage joins to the cartilage of the rib superior to it 11–12: free (floating ribs)—cartilage ends in the posterior abdominal muscles *Atypical ribs* 1st: shortest, broadest and most sharply curved true rib; contains two grooves on superior surface for the subclavian artery and vein 2nd: much longer than first rib; two facets on its head for articulation with T1 and T2 vertebral bodies 10th to 12th: only one facet on heads 11th and 12th: have no necks or tubercles Costal cartilages provide attachment for rectus abdominus; transversus abdominus; transversus thoracis; pectoralis major
Sternum	Body	Transversus thoracis; pectoralis major	Forms part of anterior thoracic wall; composed of three parts: manubrium, body, xiphoid process Longer and narrower than manubrium Has scalloped lateral borders formed by costal notches for articulation with costal cartilages Lies at level of T3 and T4 vertebral bodies
	Manubrium	–	Clavicular notch: articulates with sternal end of clavicle Lateral border: articulates with costal cartilage of 1st rib (inferior to clavicular notch) Sternal angle (of Louis): joint between manubrium and body of sternum—landmark at level of 2nd intercostal space and IV disc of T4 and T5 vertebrae
	Xiphoid process	Diaphragm; transversus thoracis; rectus abdominus	Smallest part of sternum Lies at level of T10 vertebra; midline marker for superior level of liver, central tendon of diaphragm and inferior cardiac border

The vertebral column consists of 24 bones (excluding the sacrum and coccyx). This includes 7 cervical vertebrae (covered in the head and neck section), 12 thoracic vertebrae and 5 lumbar vertebrae. The structural characteristics of these bones differ with their position in the vertebral column.

The bones of the thorax are the sternum and ribs. There are 12 pairs of ribs and the sternum is made up of three bones which become fused in later life. As well as protecting the structures within the thorax, the ribcage also provides protection for those organs in the superior regions of the abdomen.

The significant features and muscle attachments of these bones are detailed in the tables above and the anatomical arrangement illustrated in the images and sketches below.

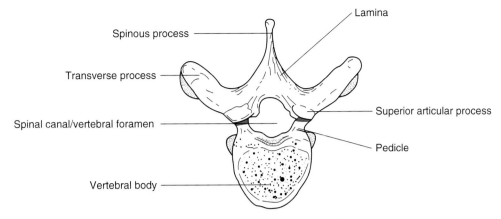

Figure 1 Typical thoracic vertebra (superior view).

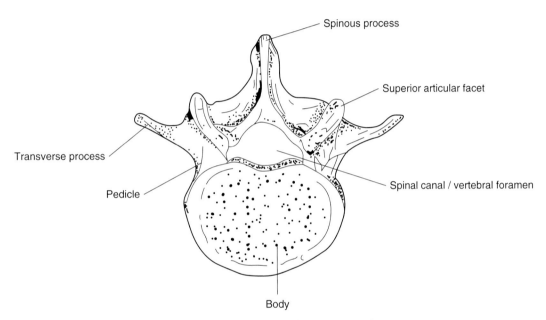

Figure 2 Typical lumbar vertebra (superior view).

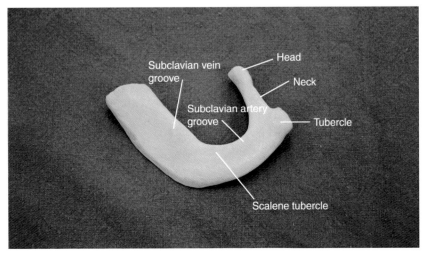

Figure 3 First rib.

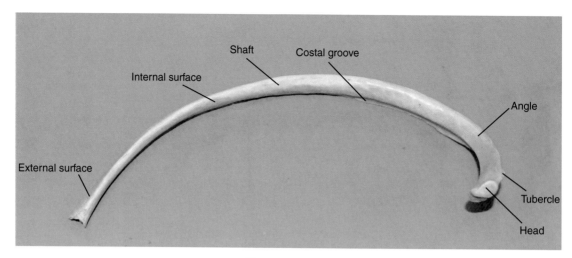

Figure 4 Typical rib.

The muscles of the back allow connection of the vertebrae with the ribs, pelvis and skull as well as with each other. They allow movement of the vertebral column, ribs and head. They also share the role of the skeleton in providing support for the body's weight and allowing movement of the trunk. Due to this role, it is quite common for some individuals to experience back pain caused by the stresses and strains on the muscles, particularly in the lower back.

The muscles of the thorax enable us to perform the act of breathing, one of the most important functions of the thorax.

The coordinated contraction and relaxation of these muscles allows the necessary volume changes in the thorax for this function to take place.

The abdominal muscles protect those structures in the more inferior regions of the abdomen as well as assisting with breathing.

The actions of each muscle, along with its attachments and innervations, are detailed in the tables below. The anatomical arrangements are illustrated in the images and sketches below.

Table 2 Muscles of the Core

Muscle	Proximal attachment	Distal attachment	Action	Innervation
Thorax				
Pectoral region				
Pectoralis major	Medial half of clavicle, anterior surface of sternum, costal cartilages of ribs 1–6 and aponeurosis of external oblique muscle	Lateral lip of bicipital groove of humerus	Flexion, adduction and medial rotation of arm	Lateral and medial pectoral nerves (C5–T1)
Pectoralis minor	Outer surfaces of ribs 3–5	Coracoid process of scapula	Protraction of scapula Depression of shoulder tip	Medial pectoral nerve (C8, T1)
Subclavius	Junction between 1st rib and costal cartilage	Groove on inferior surface of middle of clavicle	Medial movement of clavicle to stabilise sternoclavicular joint	Nerve to subclavius (C5, C6)
Thoracic wall				
External intercostals	Inferior margin of superior rib	Superior margin of inferior rib	Superior movement of ribs Aid maintenance of intercostal space during respiration Most active during inspiration	Intercostal nerves T1–T11
Innermost intercostals	Medial edge of costal groove of superior rib	Internal aspect of superior margin of inferior rib	Aid internal intercostal muscles	Intercostal nerves T1–T11

(Continued)

Table 2 (*Continued*) Muscles of the Core

Muscle	Proximal attachment	Distal attachment	Action	Innervation
Internal intercostals	Lateral edge of costal groove of superior rib	Superior margin of inferior rib deep to the insertion point of the related external intercostal	Inferior movement of ribs Aid maintenance of intercostal space during respiration Most active during expiration	Intercostal nerves T1–T11
Levatores costarum	Short-paired muscles arising from transverse processes of C7 to T11	Rib inferior to origin between tubercle and angle	Elevation of ribs	Dorsal primary rami of C8–T11 nerves
Serratus anterior	Outer surface of ribs 1–8/9	Medial border of scapula (costal surface)	Protraction of scapula Assists in rotation of scapula	Long thoracic nerve (C5–C7)
Subcostales	Internal surface (near angle) of lower ribs	Internal surface of second or third rib below	Depression of ribs	Related intercostal nerves
Transversus thoracis	Inferior aspect of deep surface of body of sternum, xiphoid process and costal cartilages of ribs 4–7	Inferior margins and internal surfaces of costal cartilages of ribs 2–6	Weak depression of ribs	Related intercostal nerves
Diaphragm	Central tendon of diaphragm	Sternal part: posterior surface of xiphoid process; costal margin; medial and lateral arcuate ligaments and L1–L3	Chief muscle of inspiration Increases thoracic cavity volume	Phrenic nerves (C3–C5)

Abdomen

Anterior abdominal wall

Muscle	Proximal attachment	Distal attachment	Action	Innervation
External oblique	Outer surfaces of the lower eight ribs (ribs 5 to 12)	Linea alba; pubic tubercle; lateral lip of iliac crest	Compression of abdominal contents Flexion and rotation of trunk	Anterior rami of T7 to T12 nerves
Internal oblique	Thoracolumbar fascia; anterior 2/3 of iliac crest; lateral 2/3 of inguinal ligament	Inferior border of the lower three or four ribs; linea alba; pubic crest and pecten pubis	Compression of abdominal contents Flexion and rotation of trunk	Anterior rami of T7 to T12 and L1 nerves
Pyramidalis	Pubis and pubic symphysis	Linea alba	Tenses linea alba	Anterior ramus of T12
Rectus abdominis	Pubic crest, pubic tubercle and pubic symphysis	Costal cartilages of ribs 5 to 7; xiphoid process	Compression of abdominal contents Flexion of trunk Stabilisation and control of pelvic tilt	Anterior rami of T7 to T12 nerves
Transversus abdominis	Thoracolumbar fascia; iliac crest; lateral 1/3 of inguinal ligament; costal cartilages of ribs 7 to 12	Linea alba; pubic crest and pecten pubis	Compression of abdominal contents	Anterior rami of T7 to T12 and L1 nerves

Posterior abdominal wall

Muscle	Proximal attachment	Distal attachment	Action	Innervation
Psoas minor	Bodies of T12 and L1 vertebrae	Pecten pubis and iliopubic eminence	Weak flexion of lumbar vertebral column	Anterior ramus of L1
Quadratus lumborum	Transverse processes of L5 vertebra; iliolumbar ligament and iliac crest	Inferior border of 12th rib; transverse processes of L1–L4 vertebrae	Lateral flexion of the trunk Stabilisation of 12th rib during inspiration	Anterior rami of T12–L4

(*Continued*)

Table 2 (*Continued*) Muscles of the Core

Muscle	Proximal attachment	Distal attachment	Action	Innervation
Back				
Intermediate				
Serratus posterior inferior	Spinous processes of T11–L3 and supraspinous ligaments	Ribs 9–12, just lateral to their angles	Depression of ribs 9–12 (probably mainly proprioceptive)	Anterior rami of T9 to T12 nerves
Serratus posterior superior	Ligamentum nuchae, spinous processes of C7–T3 and supraspinous ligaments	Ribs 2–5, lateral to their angles	Elevation of ribs 2–5 (probably mainly proprioceptive)	Anterior rami of T2 to T5 nerves
Suboccipital group				
Obliquus capitis inferior	Bifid spinous process of C2	Transverse process of vertebra C1	Rotation of head	Posterior primary ramus of C1
Obliquus capitis superior	Transverse process of vertebra C1	Occipital bone between superior and inferior nuchal lines	Extension and lateral flexion of head	Posterior primary ramus of C1
Rectus capitis posterior major	Spinous process of vertebra C2	Lateral part of inferior nuchal line of occipital bone	Extension and rotation of head	Posterior primary ramus of C1
Rectus capitis posterior minor	Posterior tubercle of posterior arch of vertebra C1	Medial part of inferior nuchal line of occipital bone	Weak extension of head	Posterior primary ramus of C1
Intrinsic/deep group				
Superficial layer				
Splenius (capitis and cervicis)	Nuchal ligament and spinous process of C7–T3 or T4 vertebrae	Splenius capitis: mastoid process; lateral third of superior nuchal line Splenius cervicis: transverse processes of C1–C3 or C4 vertebrae	Acting alone: Lateral flexion of neck and rotation of head to side of active muscles Acting together: extension of head and neck	Posterior rami of spinal nerves
Intermediate layer				
Erector spinae group				
Iliocostalis	Posterior surface of sacrum and iliac crest, spinous processes of lumbar vertebrae and L4–L5; angles of ribs 3–12	Lumborum, thoracis, cervicis—angles of ribs and transverse processes of cervical vertebrae	Acting bilaterally: extend vertebral column and head; control movement in flexion of vertebral column Acting unilaterally: laterally flex vertebral column	Posterior rami of spinal nerves
Longissimus	Transverse processes of T1–T4/T5 and lumbar vertebrae; articular processes of C4/C5–C7	Thoracis, cervicis, capitis – transverse processes of thoracic vertebrae and C2–C6; ribs 3/4–12; posterior margin of mastoid process	–	–
Spinalis	Spinous processes of T10/T11–L2; ligamentum nuchae and C7 spinous process; transverse processes of C7–T12	Thoracis, cervicis, capitis–spinous processes in the upper thoracic region (T1–T8) and C2 and to cranium	–	–

(*Continued*)

Table 2 (*Continued*) Muscles of the Core

Muscle	Proximal attachment	Distal attachment	Action	Innervation
Deep layer				
Transverso-spinalis • Multifidus • Rotatores (brevis and longus) • Semispinalis	Transverse processes Multifidus: posterior sacrum, posterior superior iliac spine, aponeurosis of erector spinae, sacroiliac ligaments, mamillary processes of lumbar vertebrae, transverse processes of T1–T3, articular processes of C4–C7 Rotatores: transverse processes of thoracic vertebrae; mamillary processes of lumbar vertebrae; articular processes of cervical vertebrae; best developed in thoracic region Semispinalis capitis: C7, T1–T6/T7; articular processes of C4–C6 Semispinalis cervicis: upper 5/6 thoracic vertebrae Semispinalis thoracis: C4 to T12 vertebrae	Spinous processes of more superior vertebrae Rotatores: spinous processes of cervical, thoracic and lumbar vertebrae Semispinalis: thoracis, cervicis, capitis—spinous processes of C2–C7 and T1–T4; occipital bone Multifidus: thickest in lumbar region; spinous processes from C2–L5	Bilaterally: extension of the vertebral column Unilaterally: rotation of trunk in opposite direction Multifidus: stabilises vertebrae during local movements of vertebral column Rotatores: stabilise vertebrae and assist local extension and rotatory movements of vertebral column; may function as organs of proprioception Semispinalis: extends head and extends and contralaterally rotates thoracic and cervical regions of vertebral column	Posterior rami of spinal nerves
Minor deep layer				
Interspinales	Spinous processes of cervical and lumbar vertebrae	Inferior surfaces of spinous processes of superior vertebrae	Aid in extension of vertebral column	Posterior rami of spinal nerves
Intertransversarii	Transverse processes of cervical and lumbar vertebrae	Transverse processes of adjacent vertebrae	Aid in lateral flexion of vertebral column Stabilise vertebral column acting bilaterally	Posterior and anterior rami of spinal nerves

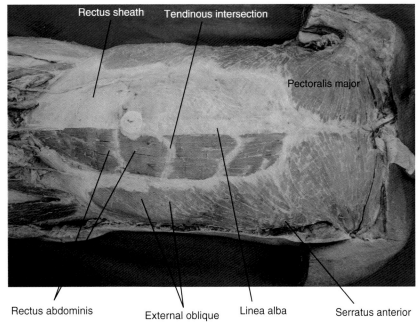

Figure 5 Abdominal muscles.

As well as joints between adjacent vertebrae in the vertebral column, there are also joints between the vertebrae and the ribs. The joints of the vertebral column allow movement, while those with the ribs anchor the ribs posteriorly facilitating movement during breathing.

Additionally, some of the ribs articulate anteriorly with sternum, while others articulate with each other via the costal cartilages.

The type and articulations of each joint, along with its action and important features, are detailed in the tables below.

Table 3 Joints of the Core

Joint	Type	Articulations	Action	Important features
Back				
Costotransverse	Synovial gliding (plane)	Tubercle of rib Transverse process of corresponding vertebra	Slight gliding	Helps control movement of the ribs to allow them to remain parallel during respiration Joint does not exist at 11th and 12th ribs
Costovertebral	Synovial plane	Head of rib Demifacets in body of corresponding thoracic vertebra and vertebra superior to it	"Pump-handle" movement—raising and lowering of ribs 2–6 "Bucket-handle" movement—raising and lowering middle of rib at ribs 7–10	1st, 11th and 12th ribs articulate only with corresponding vertebral body
Intervertebral	Secondary cartilaginous or symphysis	Adjacent vertebrae via intervertebral disc	Limited movement between successive vertebrae which when summed over the whole length of the vertebral column permits a considerable degree of flexibility	Discs are important shock absorbers between vertebrae
Zygaphophyseal	Synovial	Superior and inferior articular processes of vertebrae	Thoracic: rotation while limiting flexion and extension Lumbar: limited flexion and extension, rotation resisted	Thoracic: vertical orientation Lumbar: curved articular surfaces with interlocking processes
Thorax				
Costochondral	Primary cartilaginous or synchondrosis (connecting medium is hyaline cartilage)	Costal cartilage Sternal end of ribs	No movement at these joints in normal circumstances	–
Interchondral	Synovial gliding (plane)	Formed by costal cartilages of 6–7th, 7–8th and 8–9th ribs	Slight gliding	Joint between cartilage of ribs 9 and 10 is fibrous
Manubriosternal	Secondary cartilaginous or symphysis	Manubrium Body of sternum	None	Often ossifies in old age
Sternoclavicular	Synovial saddle joint	Medial end of clavicle Manubrium, 1st costal cartilage	Functionally a ball-and-socket joint Protraction, retraction, elevation and depression of clavicle	Separated into two compartments by an articular disc Involved in movements of shoulder girdle
Sternocostal	Primary cartilaginous joint (synchondrosis) at rib 1; synovial from ribs 2–7	Costal cartilage Sternum	Slight gliding	–
Xiphisternal	Synchondrosis	Body of sternum Xiphoid process	No significant movement at this joint	The cartilage usually ossifies with age

The ligaments of the core serve mainly to strengthen and stabilise joints and to provide points of muscular attachment.

The attachments and functions of each ligament are detailed in the tables below.

Table 4 Ligaments of the Core

Ligament	Attachments	Function
Spine		
Alar ligaments of dens	Dens of C2 Occipital condyles	Restrict excessive rotation of head
Anterior longitudinal	Base of skull Anterior surface of sacrum	Runs anterior to vertebrae; prevents hyperextension of spine; prevents one vertebra moving forward over another
Cruciform	Horizontal and longitudinal bands	Stabilises joint between dens and anterior arch of atlas; stabilises the occipitoatlantoaxial complex
Interspinous	Pass between adjacent vertebral spinous processes From base to apex of each spinous process	Prevents excessive rotation
Ligamentum flavum	Passes between laminae of adjacent vertebrae	Resists separation of laminae in flexion, assist in extension back to anatomical position
Ligamentum nuchae	External occipital protuberance and foramen magnum Spinous processes of cervical vertebrae	Supports head, resists flexion, provides muscle attachments, permits greater degree of extension
Posterior longitudinal	Posterior surfaces of vertebral bodies Lines anterior surface of vertebral canal	Resists flexion of spine
Supraspinous	Tips of spinous processes from vertebra C7 Sacrum	Limits flexion of vertebral column
Transverse ligament of atlas (horizontal band of cruciform ligament)	Extends between tubercles of medial surfaces of C1	Stabilises joint between dens and anterior arch of atlas
Abdomen		
Inguinal	Anterior superior iliac spine Pubic tubercle	Forms most inferior part of external oblique aponeurosis/floor of the inguinal canal
Lacunar	Inguinal ligament Superior pubic ramus	Medial boundary of subinguinal space—expanded medial end of the inguinal ligament
Medial arcuate	Sides of vertebrae L1 and L2 Transverse process of L1	Point of origin for some of the muscular components of the diaphragm
Lateral arcuate	Transverse process of vertebra L1 12th rib	Point of origin for some of the muscular components of the diaphragm
Thorax		
Costotransverse	Neck of rib Transverse process	Strengthens anterior aspects of joint
Lateral costotransverse	Tubercle of rib Tip of transverse process	Strengthens posterior aspects of joint
Superior costotransverse	Crest of neck of rib Transverse process superior to it	Limits movement of joint to slight gliding
Intra-articular	Crest of head of rib Intervertebral disc	Stabilises the costovertebral joints; limits movement of the rib
Sternocostal	Costal cartilages Anterior and posterior surfaces of sternum	Stabilises attachment of ribs to sternum; limits rib movement

CLINICAL SCENARIOS

Vertebral Column

Adolescent Idiopathic Scoliosis
A 14-year-old girl has been referred to the orthopaedic clinic with a 2-month history of back pain and uncharacteristic gait secondary to difference in leg length. She reports that her clothes "don't seem to fit properly anymore". On examination, the right shoulder appears to be positioned higher than the left, and on flexion of the spine, the right ribcage becomes more prominent. The history reveals that there is a family history of progressive scoliosis on the mother's side. You decide to order an X-ray and seek the advice of your seniors as to what treatment would be most beneficial in this case.

Key Findings

- It is vital to treat progressive scoliosis as it can lead to severe deformity and significant pathophysiological changes.
- The rotation of the spine can cause cardiopulmonary compromise due to ribcage deformity.
- If the curvature of the spine does not exceed 40 degrees by time the patient reaches skeletal maturity, there is a possibility that the progression may stop.
- X-rays can be used to measure the Cobb angle (angle of the curvature) and look for Risser's sign (skeletal maturation sign detected by looking at the iliac crest fusion with the pelvis).
- Non-surgical treatments such as braces are aimed at those with curvatures less than 40°.
- Surgical treatments include implanting screws and rods in order to straighten the spine and allow skeletal maturity to be reached without progression of scoliosis; the approach to surgical technique depends upon size, extent and location of scoliosis.

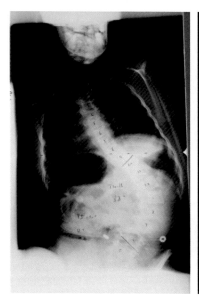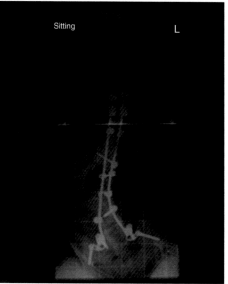

Figure 6   Severe idiopathic adolescent scoliosis: Pre- and post-operative X-rays.

Kyphosis: Spontaneous Kyphotic Collapse

A 41-year-old man has come to A&E with a 7-week history of moderate to severe neck pain. He is an IV drug user with no recorded significant medical history. He has been staying with a friend for the last 2 months after sleeping rough for a period of 2–3 years. He denies trauma to the neck.

On examination, there is point tenderness around C2 and on movement of the neck as well as clear kyphosis of the cervical spine; all other aspects of the physical examination are unremarkable. You order an MRI to confirm your suspicions of disc degeneration. You try to consent the patient for the imaging procedure but he refuses and discharges himself. He returns 6 weeks later, complaining of worsening neck pain and inability to move his neck. You repeat the examinations: he is now pyrexial and has severe point tenderness over C2 and C4, his neck movements are severely impaired and there is a palpable gap between C3 and C4 spinous processes. His WCC is high and an X-ray reveals the collapse of C3. The MRI shows an abscess near C3 region, a kyphotic angle of 80 degrees and there is evidence of osteomyelitis at C2 to C5.

Key Findings

- IV drug users have a higher risk of cervical osteomyelitis as they use the jugular vein for injection and risk introduction of bacteria both into the blood stream and directly to the periosteum.
- X-rays are useful tools in diagnosing kyphosis but are less effective in showing the cause of the deformity, for instance, osteomyelitis in this case.
- CT scans are also useful in showing deformities and abscesses but less useful for determining the cause.

Lumbar Spine Fracture

A 28-year-old man is brought to A&E following a fall from a first floor window. He is a window cleaner and was leaning out of the window when he lost his balance and fell backwards landing on the lawn of the back garden. On arrival, he was alert and cooperative with a GCS of 15; he tells you that he heard a crack, "the kind you hear when stretching your back, but louder". On examination, there was evidence of some minor abrasions on his hands and buttock area as well as pain in the lower back region that is exacerbated by movement. Examination of his spine revealed swelling in the lumbar region around the level of L1–L2 without skin laceration; pain is elicited on palpation but there was no evidence of any neurological damage in lower extremities. X-ray and CT reveal a stable lumbar wedge fracture at L1.

Key Findings
- There are different classifications for vertebral fractures. The most commonly used classification is Denis; this classification divides the spine into three columns and fractures of each column are described as either stable or unstable.
- The three column model:
  - The spine is divided into three columns.
  - The anterior column consists of the anterior longitudinal ligament and the anterior region of the vertebral body.
  - The posterior column includes the supraspinous ligament, facet joints and the pedicles.
  - The middle column comprises the posterior longitudinal ligament and the posterior vertebral body region.
- Fracture types:
  - Wedge fracture—due to vertical compression and forced flexion of the spine leading to a stable fracture. The X-ray would show a small anterior region fracture.
  - Burst fracture—due to axial force leading to shattering of the vertebral body; an unstable fracture that can lead to bone fragments protruding into the spinal canal.
  - Chance fracture—due to sudden hyperflexion of the spine; an unstable fracture also known as seat belt fracture.
  - Fracture dislocation—dislocation and fracture occur at the same time; this is also unstable and permanent stiffness can result.
- Generally, if only the anterior column is affected, the fracture is said to be stable and can be treated conservatively; any other combinations would lead to an unstable fracture that will require surgical intervention.

Spondylolysis/Pars Fracture

A 15-year-old semi-professional female gymnast is brought to your GP clinic by her mother with a 2–3 week history of back pain. The young athlete tells you that she has been training since she was 5 years old and intensively for the last 2 month to prepare herself for an upcoming competition in Berlin in 3 weeks. She says that for the last couple of weeks, she has felt a dull ache in her lower back when "bending backwards"; it subsides when resting and returns with activity. She denies any tingling or numbness in lower extremities and is quite worried about the prospect of not being well enough to prepare for the competition. She has no significant past medical history and is currently on no medication. Your examination reveals point tenderness at the level of L5, which is aggravated on extension of the spine. The rest of the examination proves unremarkable.

You order an X-ray with anterioposterior, oblique and lateral views and the results confirm your suspicions of a bilateral pars fracture. There is no evidence of spondylolisthesis.

Key Findings
- Spondylolysis is the fracture of the posterior region of the vertebra (fracture of pars interarticularis region)
- Pars fracture is a stress fracture that occurs in young athletes due to repetitive stress of the lower vertebrae; it commonly affects the 5th lumbar vertebra
- Spondylolisthesis occurs when the fracture leads to bone-weakening and shifting of the vertebra out of position
- An X-ray is usually enough to confirm the diagnosis; however, if that proves inconclusive or there are neurological signs and symptoms, both a CT and an MRI can be used for further assessment
- In the case of spondylolysis, anti-inflammatory medication and complete rest can usually contain the problem and any return to activity should be gradual and follow complete remission of symptoms; physical therapy and back braces can also be recommended in some cases
- Surgical intervention may be required if there is inadequate response to conservative treatment or if there is evidence of progressing spondylolisthesis

Key Points

- To remember the innervation of the diaphragm (phrenic nerve): C3, 4, 5 keep the diaphragm alive
- Erector spinae muscles mnemonic (lateral to medial): **I Like Standing (iliocostalis, longissimus, spinalis)**
- Lateral rotators of the hip: **piece goods often go on quilts (piriformis, gemellus superior, obturator internus, gemellus inferior, obturator externus, quadratus femoris)**
- Muscles of the anterior abdominal wall: "Spare **TIRE** around the abdomen" (**t**ransversus abdominus, **i**nternal oblique, **r**ectus abdominis, **e**xternal oblique)

5 Head and neck

Harriette Spencer and Somayyeh Shahsavari

OBJECTIVES
- Bones of the Head and Neck
- Muscles of the Head and Neck
- Joint of the Head and Neck
- Clinical Scenarios
- Key Pointers

Our facial appearance is very much dependent on our cranial bone structure; more specifically, the cranium can be divided into facial skeleton and neurocranium. The latter houses the brain by creating a cavity called the cranial vault. This cavity is constructed by the joining of eight cranial bones via sutures, namely ethmoid, frontal, occipital, sphenoid, and paired parietal and temporal bones.

There are 14 facial bones, some in pairs and some singular. The inferior nasal concha, lacrimal, maxilla, nasal, palatine and zygomatic bones exist in pairs, while the mandible and vomer are single bones.

The total of 22 skull bones also give rise to smaller cavities such as the orbital fossae for the eyes, foramina which allow the passage of blood vessels and other important structure, and sinuses which are air spaces that help reduce skull weight and increase resonance.

The neck structure consists of C1–C7 cervical vertebrae, the clavicles, the hyoid bone and the manubrium—a combination of axial and appendicular skeletal structures.

Table 1a Bones of the Head

Bone	Structure	Muscle attachments	Important features
Frontal bone	Supraorbital margin	Frontalis; orbicularis oris (orbital part)	Supraorbital notch for CN V1 (supraorbital nerve) **Articulation** Parietal bone; sphenoid bone; ethmoid bone; nasal bones; lacrimal bones; maxillae; zygomatic bones
	Frontal sinus	–	–
	Orbital process	–	Forms the roof of the orbit
Temporal bone	Petrous part	–	–
	Internal acoustic meatus	–	Facial nerve (CN VII) and vestibulocochlear nerve (CN VIII) pass through
	Mastoid process	Sternocleidomastoid; digastric (posterior belly)	–
	Temporal fossa	Temporalis	–
	Squamous temporal	–	–
	External acoustic meatus	–	–
	Zygomatic process	–	–
	Carotid canal	–	Internal carotid passes through
	Foramen lacerum	–	–
	Styloid process	Stylohyoid; styloglossus	–
	Stylomastoid foramen	–	CN VII exits skull here
Maxilla	Infraorbital margin	–	–
	Infraorbital foramen	–	CN V2 (infraorbital nerve) passes through
	Alveolar process	–	Forms the teeth sockets
	Maxillary sinus	–	–
	Frontal process	Compressor nasi	–
	Canine fossa	Levator anguli oris	–
Mandible	Body	Depressor anguli oris; depressor labii inferioris; mentalis; buccinator; digastric (anterior belly); platysma	–
	Head	Lateral pterygoid	–
	Ramus	Masseter	–
	Angle	Medial pterygoid	–
	Condyle	–	Articulates with the temporal bone at the TMJ
	Coronoid process	Temporalis	–
	Mental spine	Genioglossus; geniohyoid	–
	Mylohyoid line	Mylohyoid	–
	Digastric fossa	Anterior belly of digastric	–
Occipital bone	Foramen magnum	–	Medulla oblongata passes through at this point Accessory nerve (spinal part) and vertebral arteries pass through
	Condyles	–	–
	Hypoglossal canal	–	Hypoglossal nerve passes through
	Pharyngeal tubercle	Pharyngeal constrictors	–

(Continued)

Table 1a (*Continued*) Bones of the Head

Bone	Structure	Muscle attachments	Important features
	External occipital protuberance	–	–
	Superior and inferior Nuchal lines	– Occipital belly of occipitofrontalis	– –
	Internal occipital protuberance	–	Serves as the attachment site for the meninges
Sphenoid bone	Body	–	Articulates with occipital bone
	Air spaces	–	–
	Sella turcica	–	–
	Greater wing	Lateral pterygoid	–
	Lesser wing	–	–
	Optic foramen	–	–
	Anterior and posterior clinoid processes	–	Serve as an attachment for the dura
	Superior orbital fissure	–	Lacrimal nerve, frontal nerve, nasociliary nerve (CN V1), trochlear nerve (CN IV) and abducens (CN VI) nerves pass through Superior ophthalmic vein passes through
	Foramen rotundum	–	Maxillary division of trigeminal nerve (CN V2)
	Foramen ovale	–	Mandibular division of trigeminal (CN V3), and lesser petrosal nerve pass through
	Foramen spinosum	–	Middle meningeal artery passes through
	Spine	–	Attachment for the sphenomandibular ligament
	Lateral pterygoid plates	Medial and lateral pterygoids	–
	Medial pterygoid plates	–	–
	Hamulus	–	–
Ethmoid	Crista galli	–	–
	Perpendicular plate	–	–
	Cribriform plate	–	Olfactory nerves pass through
	Ethmoid sinus	–	
	Superior turbinates	–	–
	Inferior turbinates	–	–
Zygoma	Zygomatic arch	Masseter	Articulates with the temporal bone
Parietal	Diploe	–	Articulates with: • Frontal bones; the opposite parietal bone; occipital bone; temporal bone; sphenoid bone
Vomer	–	–	–
Lacrimal bone	–	–	Articulates with: • Frontal bone; ethmoid bone; maxilla; inferior nasal concha
Inferior nasal concha	–	–	–
Palatine	Perpendicular plate Horizontal plate	–	Forms posterior part of hard palate and lateral wall of nasal cavity
Nasal bone	–	Procerus	Articulates with: • Frontal bone; ethmoid bone; the opposite nasal bone; maxilla
Hyoid bone	Greater horn, lesser horn, body	Stylohyoid; mylohyoid; geniohyoid; sternohyoid; thyrohyoid; omohyoid (superior belly); hyoglossus; middle contrictor of pharynx	The hyoid is unique in that it does not articulate with any other bones

Table 1b Bones of the Neck

Vertebrae	Body	Vertebral foramen	Transverse process	Articular process	Spinous process	Muscles attachments	Articulations
C1 (atlas)	No vertebral body No disc between C1 and C2	Bounded by anterior and posterior arches; anterior arch has facet for dens	Lateral mass with transverse foramen	Superior articular facets articulate with occipital condyles	No spinous process— posterior tubercle	Levator scapulae (C1–4) Suboccipital muscles	Connects the skull & the spine by the atlanto occipital joint Occipital condyles
C2 (axis)	Dens attached superiorly	Oval	Vertebral arteries and accompanying venous and sympathetic plexus pass through foramina, except C7 which transmits only small accessory vertebral veins; anterior and posterior tubercles	Superior articular facets permit rotation between C1 and C2	Short, bifid	–	The odontoid process allows rotation at C1
C3–6	Small and wider side to side than AP Superior surface is concave Inferior surface is convex Uncinate processes	Large and triangular		Superior facets directed supero-posteriorly; inferior facets infero-anteriorly	C3–C5 short and bifid	Trapezius Semispinalis cervicis/ capitis Scalenes Prevertebral muscles	Between vertebral bodies and articular processes Uncovertebral joints at lateral extremeties of C2–C7 vertebral bodies
C7 (vertebra prominens)	–	–	Foramen transversar- ium small or absent	–	The longest spinous process, not bifid	Rhomboid minor Splenius capitis Trapezius	–

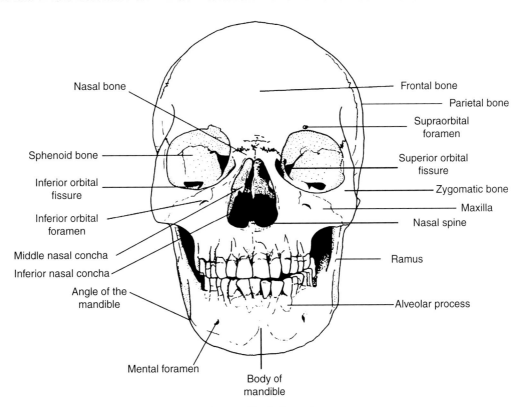

Figure 1a The skull, anterior.

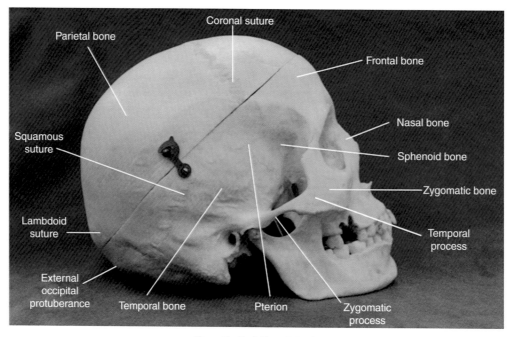

Figure 1b Skull (lateral view).

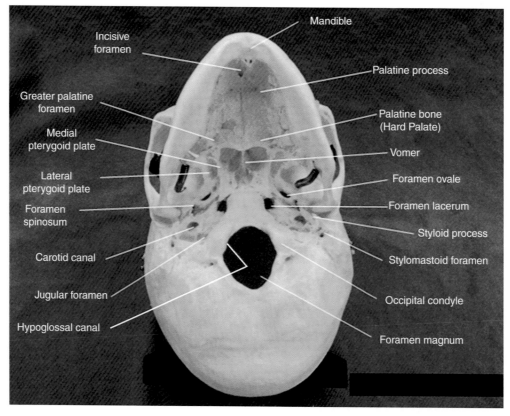

Figure 1c Skull (inferior view).

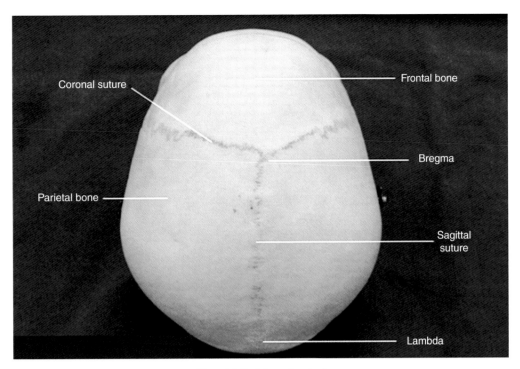

Figure 1d Skull (superior view).

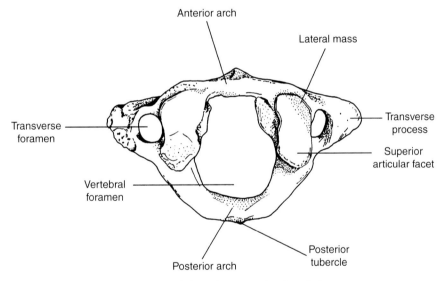

Figure 2a Cervical vertebra 1; superior view of atlas.

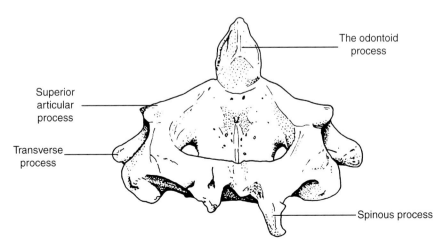

Figure 2b Cervical vertebrae 2; posterior view of the axis.

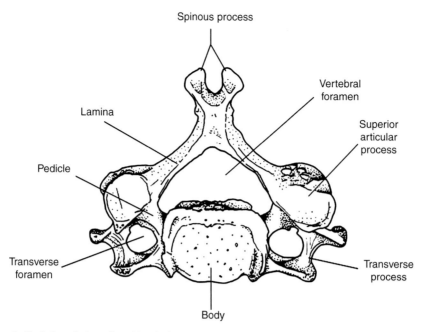

Figure 2c Typical cervical vertebrae (C3–6).The spinous processes are bifid and there is now a prominent body.

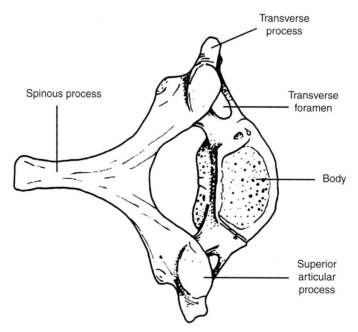

Figure 2d Cervical vertebrae 7; superior view of the vertebra prominens. The spinous process is longer than in all the other cervical vertebrae.

Muscles of the head and neck can be divided as follows:
- Anterior neck = sternohyoid, omohyoid, sternothy-roid, thyrohyoid, stylohyoid, digastric, mylohyoid and geniohyoid
- Anterolateral neck = scalenes: anterior, middle and posterior
- Superficial neck = sternocleidomastoid and platysma
- Epicranial = occipitalis and frontalis (occipitofrontalis)
- Extraocular = levator palpebrae superioris, lateral/medial/superior/inferior rectus and superior/infe-rior oblique

- Muscles of facial expression = including orbicularis oculi, corrugator supercilii, orbicularis oris, levator labii, zygomaticus minor/major, risorius, levator anguli oris, buccinator, depressor anguli oris, depres-sor labii inferioris
- Muscles of mastication = masseter, temporalis and medial/lateral pterygoids
- Prevertebral = longus colli, longus capitis and rectus capitis anterior/lateral
- Suboccipital = obliquus capitis superior/inferior and rectus capitis posterior major/minor

Table 2 Muscles of the Head and Neck

Muscle	Proximal attachment	Distal attachment	Action	Innervation
Facial muscles				
Buccinator	Alveolar process of maxilla & mandible; pterygomandibular raphe	Blends into the fibres of orbicularis oris at the angle of the mouth	Compression of cheeks Blowing and sucking actions Holds cheeks against teeth Assists in mastication	Facial nerve (buccal branches)
Depressor anguli oris	Oblique line of mandible	Angle of mouth	Pulls the angle of the mouth downwards	Facial nerve (buccal and mandibular branches)
Depressor labii inferioris	Mandible between the symphysis and mental foramen	Skin of lower lip	Draws the lower lip down and outwards	Facial nerve (mandibular branch)
Frontalis	Epicranial aponeurosis	Skin superior to supraorbital margin	Draws scalp forward Raises eyebrows Wrinkles forehead	Facial nerve (temporal branches)
Levator labii superioris	Inferior margin of orbit	Skin of the upper lip	Elevation of upper lip	Facial nerve (buccal branch)
Levator palpebrae superioris	Apex of the orbit above the optic canal; lesser wing of sphenoid	Skin and fascia of upper eyelid	Elevation of upper eyelid	Oculomotor/ sympathetic nerve
Masseter	Zygomatic arch	Ramus and coronoid process of mandible	Elevation & protraction of mandible	Trigeminal nerve (V3)
Mentalis	Anterior midline of the mandible near the mental symphysis	Skin of the chin	Elevation of skin of the chin	Facial nerve
Nasalis	Maxilla above the canine and incisor teeth	Ala of the nose	Flaring of nostrils Flattening of nose	Facial nerve (buccal branch)
Occipitalis	Occipital bone (superior nuchal line); mastoid process	Epicranial aponeurosis	Draws scalp backward Anchoring and retraction of galea posteriorly	Facial nerve (posterior auricular)
Orbicularis oculi (2 parts)	Medial orbital margin and the medial palpebral ligament (orbital part); medial palpebral ligament (palpebral part)	Skin of lateral cheek (orbital part); lateral palpebral raphe (palpebral part)	Closes the eyelids gently (palpebral part) or forcefully (orbital part) Assists the flow of the secretions of lacrimal gland	Facial nerve (temporal and zygomatic branches)
Orbicularis oris	Skin and fascia of the lips	Skin and fascia of the lips	Sphincter of mouth; pursing of lips	Facial nerve (buccal branch)
Risorius	Fascia of the cheek	Skin of the angle of the mouth (modiolus)	Draws the corner of mouth laterally	Facial nerve (buccal branches)
Temporalis	Temporal fossa and temporal fascia	Coronoid process of mandible	Elevation & retraction of mandible	Trigeminal nerve (V3)
Zygomaticus major	Upper lateral surface of zygomatic bone	Skin of the angle of the mouth	Elevation and lateral movement of corner of mouth	Facial nerve (zygomatic and buccal branches)
Zygomaticus minor	Lower surface of zygomatic bone	Lateral part of the upper lip	Elevation of upper lip	Facial nerve (buccal branch)
Neck				
Anterior belly of digastric	Digastric fossa of mandible	Body of hyoid via an intermediate tendon	Elevates hyoid bone during swallowing Depresses mandible (opens mouth)	Trigeminal nerve (V3)
Cricothyroid	Anterior and lateral portion of cricoid cartilage of larynx	Anterior inferior border and inferior horn of thyroid cartilage	Elongates and places tension on vocal cords Draws the thyroid cartilage anteriorly	Vagus nerve CN X (superior laryngeal branch)

(Continued)

Table 2 (*Continued*) Muscles of the Head and Neck

Muscle	Proximal attachment	Distal attachment	Action	Innervation
Genioglossus	Superior mental spine of mandible (symphysis menti)	Dorsum of tongue and body of hyoid	Inferior—protrude tongue Middle—Depress tongue Superior—draw the tip of the tongue back and down	Hypoglossal nerve CN XII
Geniohyoid	Inferior mental spine of the mandible (symphysis menti)	Body of the hyoid bone	Elevates the hyoid bone Depresses the mandible	C1 via the hypoglossal nerve CN XII
Hyoglossus	Hyoid bone (greater horn)	Into the intrinsic muscles on the lateral side of the tongue	Depresses the sides of the tongue Retraction of the tongue	Hypoglossal nerve CN XII
Lateral pterygoid	Lateral surface of lateral pterygoid plate; greater wing of sphenoid bone	Capsule of temporo-mandibular joint; pterygoid fovea	Protrusion, depression and lateral excursion of mandible Chewing	Trigeminal nerve (V3)
Medial pterygoid	Medial surface of lateral pterygoid plate of the sphenoid	Inner surface of mandible; angle of mandible	Protract, elevate and lateral movement of mandible	Trigeminal nerve (V3)
Mylohyoid	Inner surface of the mandible (mylohyoid line of mandible)	Body of hyoid bone and midline raphe	Elevates hyoid bone and floor of mouth Depress mandible	Nerve to mylohyoid. Trigeminal nerve (V3)
Omohyoid (2 bellies)	Suprascapular notch (inferior belly); body of hyoid (superior belly)	Clavicle via intermediate tendon	Depression, retraction and stabilisation of hyoid bone	Ansa cervicalis (C2, 3)
Platysma	Skin & fascia overlying Pectoralis major and deltoid	Inferior border of mandible; skin of the lower face	Tenses skin of neck Depression of the corners of the mouth (sad face)	Facial nerve CN VII (cervical branch)
Posterior belly of digastric	Mastoid process of temporal bone	Body of hyoid bone via intermediate tendon	Elevates hyoid bone Depresses mandible (opens mouth)	Facial nerve CN VII
Scalenus anterior	Transverse processes of cervical vertebrae 3–6	Scalene tubercle of first rib	Accessory respiratory muscle Flexion of neck Rotation of neck to opposite side	Ventral rami of cervical nerves C4–C6
Scalenus medius	Transverse processes of cervical vertebrae 2–7	Superior surface of 1st rib posteriorly to the subclavian artery	Rotation of neck to opposite side Accessory respiratory muscle	Ventral rami of cervical nerves C3–C8
Scalenus posterior	Transverse processes of cervical vertebrae 5–6	2nd rib lateral surface	Accessory respiratory muscle	Ventral rami of cervical nerves C6–C8)
Sternocleidomastoid (two heads)	Manubrium (sternal head); medial third of clavicle (clavicular head)	Mastoid process of temporal bone; lateral superior nuchal line of occipital bone	Unilaterally flexes head to the same side Rotates head to opposite side Bilaterally flexes neck Accessory respiratory muscle (inhalation)	Accessory nerve CN XI (spinal part); C2 & C3— proprioception
Sternohyoid	Medial end of clavicle and manubrium of sternum	Body of hyoid bone	Depress and stabilises hyoid after elevation	Ansa cervicalis (C1–3)
Stylohyoid	Styloid process of temporal bone	Body of hyoid bone	Elevates & retracts hyoid bone	Facial nerve CN VII
Styloglossus	Styloid process (anterior side); stylohyoid ligament	Posterolateral side of the tongue	Retraction and elevation of the tongue	Hypoglossal nerve CN XII

(*Continued*)

Table 2 (*Continued*) Muscles of the Head and Neck

Muscle	Proximal attachment	Distal attachment	Action	Innervation
Stylopharyngeus	Styloid process of temporal bone	Thyroid cartilage; pharyngeal wall	Elevates the larynx especially during swallowing	Glossopharyngeal nerve CN IX
Sternothyroid	Manubrium of sternum; first costal cartilage	Thyroid cartilage of layrnx	Depress thyroid cartilage after elevation	Ansa cervicalis (C2, C3)
Thyrohyoid	Thyroid cartilage (oblique line)	Greater horn of hyoid bone	Elevates thyroid cartilage Depresses and stabilises hyoid bone	Ansa cervicalis (C1); descending hypoglossal nerve

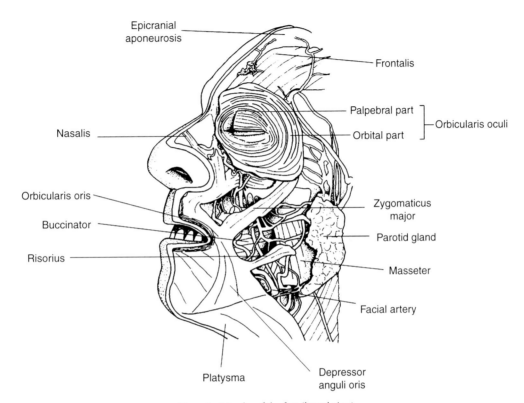

Figure 3a Muscles of the face (lateral view).

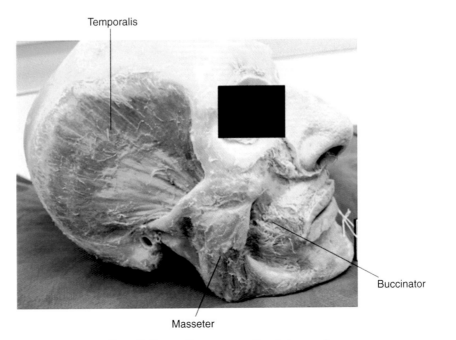

Figure 3b Temporalis, masseter and buccinator muscles.

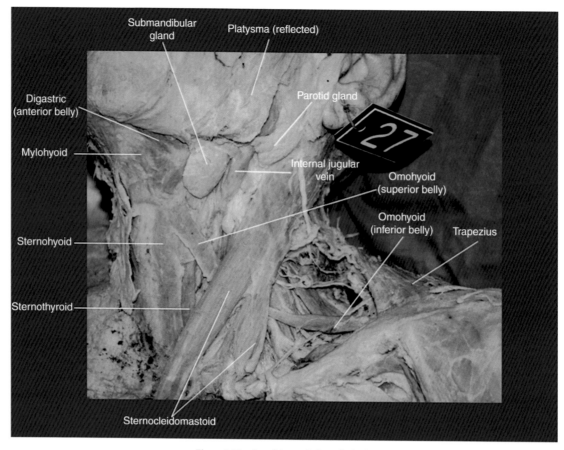

Figure 4 Muscles of the neck (lateral view).

The type and articulations of each joint, along with its action and important features, are detailed in the tables below. As mentioned in the upper limb section, a ligament is an attachment between either two bones or bone and cartilage, hence forming a joint and providing a limited range of movements at that joint. With this limitation comes greater alignment of bones and more controlled and precise movements.

The relevant neck ligaments have been included in the core section's "ligaments of the core" table.

Table 3 Joints of the Head and Neck

Joint	Type	Articulation	Action	Important features
Head				
Temporomandibular	Condyloid (synovial), with articular disc	Condylar process of the mandible Mandibular fossa of squamous part temporal bone	Protrusion Retrusion Lateral excursion (side to side) Opening and closing of the jaw	• Lateral temporomandibular ligament • Sphenomandibular ligament (medial)
Coronal suture	Fibrous	Frontal bone Parietal bone (2)	None	–
Intermaxillary suture	Fibrous	Palatine process Maxillae	None	–
Lamboidal suture	Fibrous	Occipital bone Parietal bone	None	–
Metopic suture	Neonatal suture (persists in 5–10% of adults)	Ossification centres of the frontal bones	None	–

(Continued)

Table 3 (*Continued*) Joints of the Head and Neck

Joint	Type	Articulation	Action	Important features
Sagittal suture	Fibrous	Parietal bones	None	–
Neck				
Atlanto occipital	Synovial	Occipital condyles Lateral masses of atlas	Flexion of neck (as in nodding) Extension of neck	Ligaments: anterior and posterior atlanto occipital membrane
Atlanto axial	Synovial	Odontoid process Anterior arch of atlas Also articulation between lateral masses	Rotation of head on atlas	Ligaments: apical ligament, alar ligaments, cruciform ligament
Zygapophyseal	Synovial	Articular processes of an inferior and superior vertebrae	Flexion Extension, some rotation	–

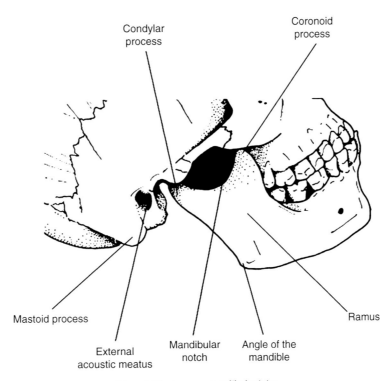

Figure 5 The temporomandibular joint.

CLINICAL SCENARIOS

Skull Fractures

Depressed Fracture

A 22-year-old man was brought to A&E following an incident of gang violence. He had been struck over the head with an axe and repeatedly attacked with a broken bottle, resulting in lacerations on his extremities. He had immediately lost consciousness after the blow to the head and remained unconscious for about 15 min; there was reportedly some nausea and vomiting in the ambulance on the way to the hospital.

On arrival, he was conscious with a GCS of 14 and was oriented with regards to time, place and person. There was an open wound about 10 × 2 cm over his right occipitoparietal skull region. A CT scan was ordered that showed a right comminuted depressed fracture of the occipitoparietal bone.

Typical Findings
- Skull fractures are either linear or depressed and depressed fractures may be open or closed.
- A depressed fracture can lead to complications such as infections and seizures and must be addressed immediately; prophylactic antibiotics and anti-seizure medication is sometimes given.
- In this type of fracture, the part of the bone that is fractured can sink below the plane of the skull and its edges can become locked under the normal contour of the surrounding bones; this can cause penetration of underlying tissue and long-lasting damage.
- It is important to note that although the fracture is palpable on examination, it may not be aligned with the scalp laceration, as the scalp is mobile. It is therefore vital that the entire cranium is examined thoroughly.

Basilar Fracture

A 32-year-old man was brought to A&E following a road traf-fic accident with a GCS of 5. He had no significant previous medical history and was on no medication. A CT scan of the head showed frontal bone contusion with no further lesions detected. He was transferred to ICU for observation and assisted ventilation; he regained consciousness within a few hours and was extubated on day 3. A thorough neurological examination was subsequently carried out that showed bilat-eral facial nerve palsy and dysphagia with an absent gag reflex. A second CT scan was carried out, which revealed skull base fracture of the temporal bone. An MRI was carried out to rule out cerebellum involvement.

Typical Findings
- This is a linear fracture at the skull base and usually involves the temporal bone.
- Cranial nerves can become trapped at the site of fracture and lead to neurological deficits on examination.
- If the sphenoid bone is involved, the intracavernous internal carotid artery can potentially form pseudoaneurysms.
- A basilar fracture can also cause a tear in the dura mater, leading to a pathway for communication between the subarachnoid space, paranasal sinuses and the middle ear that can be confirmed by CSF leaking out of the ear (CSF otorrhoea) or the nose (CSF rhinorrhoea). Most CSF leaks are self-limiting within few days.
- CT scans are not entirely effective in detecting skull base fractures and a thorough clinical examination and repeat scans are often required to make the diagnosis.

Key Points

Facial bones: **Valerie can not make my pet zebra laugh**
- **Vomer**
- **Conchae**
- **Nasal**
- **Maxilla**
- **Mandible**
- **Palatine**
- **Zygomatic**
- **Lacrimal**

Bones of the skull: **STEP OF** 6
- **Sphenoid**
- **Temporal**
- **Ethmoid**
- **Parietal**
- **Occipital**
- **Frontal**

Bones of the medial wall of the bony orbit of the eye: **My little eye sits in the orbit**
- **Maxilla**
- **Lacrimal**
- **Ethmoid**
- **Sphenoid**

Triangles of the neck:
1. Anterior triangle boundaries:
   - Anterior = median neck line
   - Posterior = anterior edge of the sternocleidomastoid
   - Superior = inferior edge of mandible
   - Apex = suprasternal notch
   - Floor = thyroid, pharynx and larynx structures
   - Roof = platysma

2. Posterior triangle boundaries:
   - Anterior = posterior edge of sternocleidomastoid
   - Posterior = anterior edge of trapezius
   - Inferior = middle one-third of clavicle
   - Apex = superior nuchal line of occipital bone

6 Test yourself! Exam-style questions

Philip James Adds and Somayyeh Shahsavari

1. A 40-year-old woman has a pleomorphic adenoma excised from her right parotid gland. Following the surgery, she finds that she is unable to close her right eye.

   Which nerve is most likely to have been damaged during the surgical procedure?

   (a) Facial nerve
   (b) Hypogolossal nerve
   (c) Lingual nerve
   (d) Ophthalmic nerve
   (e) Trigeminal nerve

2. A 35-year-old man presents to his GP complaining of occasional "lightning strikes" of pain affecting his face. The pain appears quite suddenly and unpredictably below his left eye. The GP explains that he is suffering from neuralgia affecting the sensory nerves of his face.

   Which nerve is responsible for the sensory supply to the cheek region?

   (a) Buccal branch of the facial nerve
   (b) Mandibular division of the trigeminal nerve
   (c) Maxillary division of the trigeminal nerve
   (d) Ophthalmic division of the trigeminal nerve
   (e) Zygomatic branch of the facial nerve

3. Following a fall from a bicycle, a 20-year-old woman is sent for an X-ray of her head (shown below).

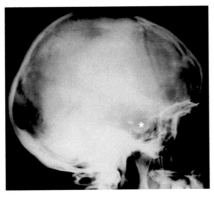

What term best describes the region indicated by the asterisk (*) in the image?

   (a) Carotid canal
   (b) Crista galli
   (c) Ethmoidal sinus
   (d) Optic canal
   (e) Pituitary fossa

4. A 60-year-old man complains to his GP of a "lump" at the back of his tongue. He is sent for an MRI scan (shown below).

   What muscle is indicated by the arrow?

   (a) Genioglossus
   (b) Geniohyoid
   (c) Hyoglossus
   (d) Palatoglossus
   (e) Styloglossus

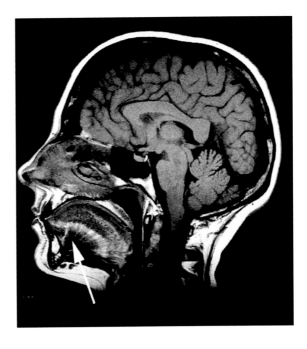

More questions/answers can be found in the online version of this publication, *Online features*.

5. During a game of football, the goalkeeper dives for the ball and hits his head on the goalpost. He is taken to A&E and a precautionary X-ray is taken (shown below).

What term best describes the bone indicated by the arrow in the image?

(a) Frontal
(b) Occipital
(c) Parietal
(d) Sphenoid
(e) Temporal

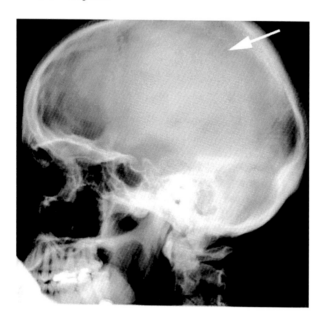

6. A patient who complains of recurrent headaches is sent for a scan (shown below).

What term best describes this type of image?

(a) CT scan
(b) PET scan
(c) T1 weighted MRI
(d) T2 weighted MRI

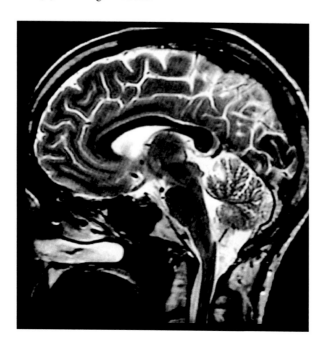

7. A 50-year-old heavy smoker complains to his GP of chest pains and shortage of breath. He is referred to a specialist for further investigations, and is sent for a CT scan.

In the image below, what term best describes the structure indicated by the arrow?

(a) Facet joint
(b) Lamina
(c) Spinous process
(d) Superior articular process
(e) Transverse process

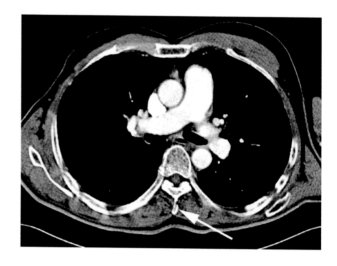

8. A 65-year-old woman is sent for a chest X-ray (shown below).

What term best describes the feature indicated by the arrow?

(a) Breast shadow
(b) Costodiaphragmatic recess
(c) Oblique fissure
(d) Parietal pleura
(e) Transverse fissue

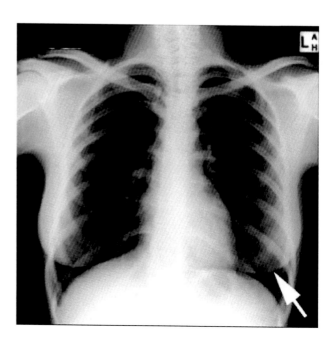

9. A 75-year-old man complaining of pain on passing water and haematuria is sent for a CT scan (below).

   What term best describes the structure indicated by the arrow in the image?

   (a) Iliacus
   (b) Obturator externus
   (c) Obturator internus
   (d) Psoas major
   (e) Urinary bladder

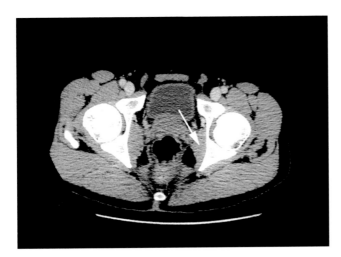

10. A patient complaining of abdominal pain is sent for a CT scan (shown below).

    What term best describes the structure indicated by the arrow?

    (a) Crus of diaphragm
    (b) Erector spinae
    (c) Fundus of stomach
    (d) Latissimus dorsi
    (e) Trapezius

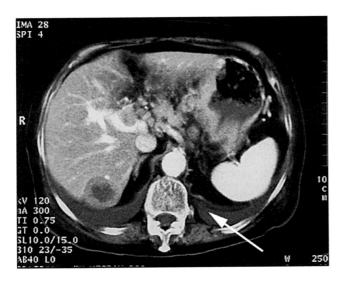

11. You are inserting a chest drain into a patient with pleural effusion.

    What phrase best applies to the location of the intercostal neurovascular bundle?

    (a) Just above the rib between the external and internal intercostal muscles
    (b) Just above the rib between the internal and innermost intercostal muscles
    (c) Just below the rib between the external and internal intercostal muscles
    (d) Just below the rib between the internal and innermost intercostal muscles
    (e) Just below the rib superficial to the external intercostal muscles

12. A student suffers a painful knee injury during a game of rugby. He is referred to an orthopaedic clinic and sent for an MRI scan (show below).

    What term best describes the structure indicated by the arrow?

    (a) Anterior cruciate ligament
    (b) Lateral collateral ligament
    (c) Medial collateral ligament
    (d) Oblique popliteal ligament
    (e) Posterior cruciate ligament

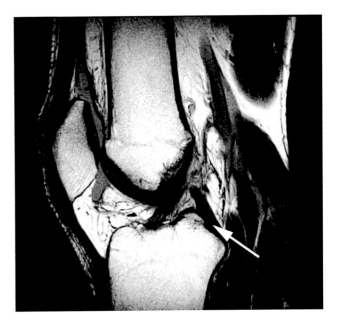

13. A 75-year-old woman with painful hips is sent for an X-ray (shown below).

What term best describes the muscle that attaches at the point indicated by the arrow?

(a) Iliopsoas
(b) Pectineus
(c) Rectus femoris
(d) Sartorius
(e) Vastus medialis

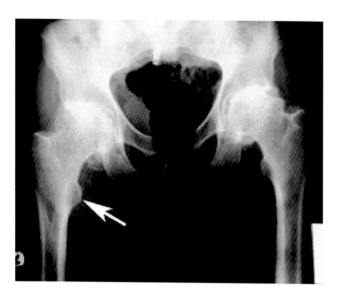

14. A teenage boy attends A&E complaining that he is unable to move his head following a tackle in a game of rugby. You carry out a full examination and conclude that he has torn his right sternocleidomastoid muscle.

Which of the following best describes the nerve supply to this muscle?

(a) Accessory nerve
(b) Axillary nerve
(c) Facial nerve
(d) First intercostal nerve
(e) Supraclavicular nerve

15. You are examining a 60-year-old man who complains of headaches and facial pain, especially when opening and closing his mouth, and when chewing. You suspect TMJ disorder.

What nerve gives motor supply to the muscles of mastication?

(a) Facial nerve
(b) Hypoglossal nerve
(c) Lingual nerve
(d) Spinal accessory nerve
(e) Trigeminal nerve

16. Following a fall from a bicycle, a 20-year-old woman is sent for an X-ray of her head (shown below).

What term best describes the region indicated by the arrow in the image?

(a) Carotid canal
(b) Crista galli
(c) Ethmoidal sinus
(d) Frontal sinus
(e) Piuitary fossa

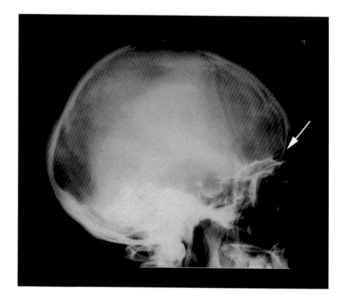

17. A 25-year-old motorcyclist is brought into A&E by ambulance following a head on collision with a parked tractor on a country road. You observe that there is abnormal posterior subluxation of the tibia on the femur.

Which of the following ligaments is most likely to have been ruptured?

(a) Anterior cruciate
(b) Lateral collateral
(c) Medial collateral
(d) Meniscofemoral
(e) Posterior cruciate

18. A 50-year-old woman presents with pain, tingling and numbness in her wrist and hand affecting the thumb, index, middle and lateral half of the ring finger. The pain is worse at night and in the morning. She has positive Tinel's sign and Phalen's test and there are signs of thenar wasting.

Which one of the following is the most likely nerve affected?

(a) Axillary
(b) Median
(c) Musculocutaneous
(d) Radial
(e) Ulnar

19. A 24-year-old rugby player presents to A&E with an acutely painful shoulder. He fell on his outstretched arm during a match. On examination, there is a "lump" anterior to the right shoulder. During the examination, the patient resists any form of movement in the shoulder.

What is the most likely diagnosis of his injury?

(a) Clavicle fracture
(b) Complete rotator cuff tear
(c) Dislocated acromioclavicular joint
(d) Dislocated glenohumeral joint
(e) Fractured proximal humerus

20. A 35-year-old judo enthusiast suffers an anterior dislocation of the shoulder joint. He presents to A&E where he is assessed by a surgical registrar who notes an area of anaesthesia over the insertion of the deltoid muscle ("regimental badge" area) both before and after reduction of the dislocation.

Which of the following shoulder muscles is most likely to exhibit paralysis in this patient?

(a) Infraspinatus
(b) Subscapularis
(c) Supraspinatus
(d) Teres minor
(e) Trapezius

21. A 25-year-old man who survived being stabbed in the neck 3 weeks earlier presents to you with weakness of the ipsilateral shoulder. He is unable to abduct his arm beyond 90° or shrug his shoulder.

Which of the following muscles is most likely to be paralysed?

(a) Latissimus dorsi
(b) Pectoralis major
(c) Subscapularis
(d) Teres major
(e) Trapezius

22. A 25-year-old man presents to A&E after falling off his motorcycle and landing on his right shoulder. You observe that he has a bruise over his right acromion and his right upper limb is adducted at the shoulder, extended at the elbow, with the forearm pronated. He is unable to abduct his arm.

Which of the following parts of his brachial plexus is most likely injured?

(a) Lower trunk
(b) Medial cord
(c) Middle trunk
(d) Posterior cord
(e) Upper trunk

23. A 35-year-old woman with an aggressive breast carcinoma undergoes a modified radical mastectomy. She presents to you 6 weeks post-operatively complaining of weakness in the ipsilateral upper limb. You examine her and find that she has significant winging of the ipsilateral scapula.

Which of the following nerves is most likely to have been injured in the mastectomy?

(a) Long thoracic
(b) Median
(c) Musculocutaneous
(d) Thoracodorsal
(e) Upper subscapular

24. A 25-year-old woman is brought into A&E by ambulance following a collision in a game of hockey. You observe that her right knee is swollen and painful. After administration of morphine for the pain, you examine the knee further and find that there is abnormal anterior movement of the tibia on the femur (a positive anterior drawer test).

Which of the following ligaments is most likely to be ruptured?

(a) Anterior cruciate
(b) Lateral collateral
(c) Medial collateral
(d) Meniscofemoral
(e) Posterior cruciate

25. Following a fall from a motorbike, a 20-year-old man with a suspected cranial fracture is sent for an X-ray (shown below).

What type of joint is indicated by the arrow?

(a) Fibrous
(b) Primary cartilaginous
(c) Secondary cartilaginous
(d) Symphysis
(e) Synovial

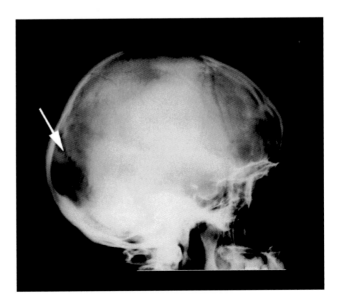

26. A 20-year-old student attends his GP surgery with a painful soft swelling on the point of his elbow. His doctor diagnoses bursitis, and sends him for an X-ray (shown below).

    Which term best describes the action on the elbow joint of the muscle that attaches at the point indicated by the arrowhead?

    (a) Extension
    (b) Flexion
    (c) Pronation
    (d) Rotation
    (e) Supination

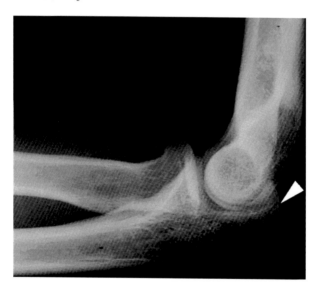

27. A 50-year old man with suspected lumbar disc herniation is sent for a CT scan (shown below).

    What term best describes the nerve supply to the muscles indicated by the arrow?

    (a) Lumbosacral plexus
    (b) Intercostal nerves
    (c) Sciatic nerve
    (d) Segmental supply by dorsal primary rami
    (e) Segmental supply by ventral primary rami

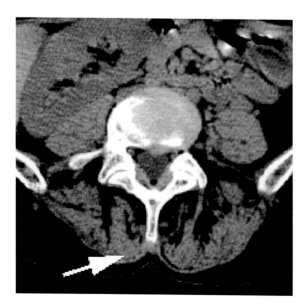

28. Following a traffic accident, a 60-year-old woman is suspected of suffering a rib fracture and is sent for a chest X-ray (shown below).

    What term best describes the type of joint indicated by the arrow?

    (a) Condylar
    (b) Hinge
    (c) Pivot
    (d) Plane
    (e) Saddle

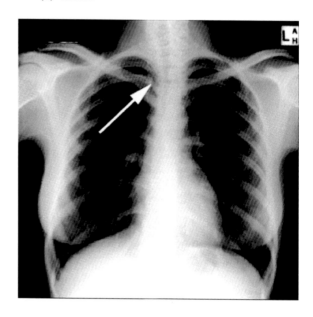

29. A young man attends A&E after receiving a superficial knife wound below his axilla during a disturbance outside a nightclub. On examination, you observe that his scapula on the injured side is protruding from his posterior chest wall ("winging" of the scapula).

    Which muscle is chiefly responsible for maintaining the position of the scapula against the chest wall?

    (a) Deltoid
    (b) Levator scapulae
    (c) Rhomboid major
    (d) Serratus anterior
    (e) Trapezius

30. A patient presents to his GP for a follow-up appointment 3 months after a fracture of the head of the right fibula. The GP notices that the patient walks with ipsilateral foot drop and an exaggerated right knee lift. The GP suspects paralysis of the ankle dorsiflexors.

    Which nerve supplies the ankle dorsiflexors?

    (a) Deep peroneal (fibular)
    (b) Femoral
    (c) Sural
    (d) Superficial peroneal (fibular)
    (e) Tibial

31. A 66-year-old retired teacher presents with lower back pain, and pain radiating down her right leg. She says she has been busy digging the garden.

    What is the most likely cause of her symptoms?

    (a) Anterior displacement of the L3/L4 intervertebral disc
    (b) Fracture of the right inferior articular process of L1
    (c) Inflammation of the uncovertebral joints
    (d) Posterolateral herniation of the L4/L5 intervertebral disc
    (e) Posterior herniation of the L1/L2 intervertebral disc

32. A 19-year-old student attends A&E following a scuffle outside a club in which he was attacked with a knife. He had held his arm up to protect his face, but had been cut on the chest wall below his right axilla. On examination, he was found to be unable to protract his shoulder on the injured side.

    Which muscle is responsible for protraction of the scapula?

    (a) Biceps brachii
    (b) Levator scapulae
    (c) Pectoralis major
    (d) Serratus anterior
    (e) Trapezius

33. A 25-year-old woman is brought to A&E following a heavy fall from a trampoline. She complains of back pain, and you send her for a lumbar X-ray.

    In the image below, what term best describes the type of joint indicated by the arrow?

    (a) Fibrous
    (b) Primary cartilaginous
    (c) Secondary cartilaginous
    (d) Syndesmosis
    (e) Synovial

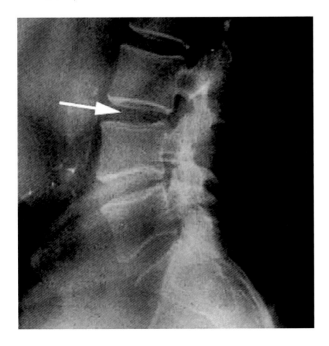

34. A 60-year-old man complains of lower back pain. His GP sends him for an X-ray (below).

    What term best describes the structure indicated by the arrow?

    (a) Inferior articular process
    (b) Lamina
    (c) Pedicle
    (d) Spinous process
    (e) Transverse process

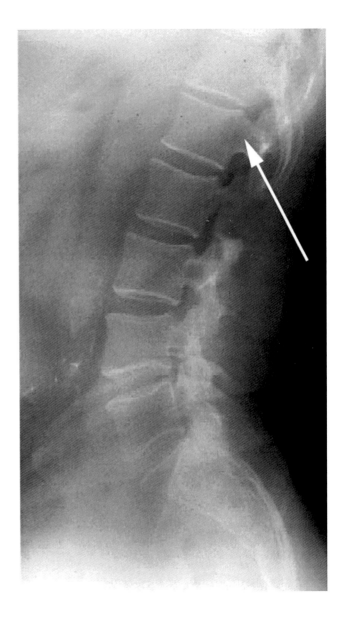

35. (Continued from Q. 34) His GP explains that his pain is caused by a "slipped disc" pressing on a nerve. The affected nerve emerges between the fourth and fifth lumbar vertebrae.

    What term best describes this nerve?

    (a) L4 dorsal primary ramus
    (b) L4 mixed spinal nerve
    (c) L4 motor root
    (d) L4 sensory root
    (e) L4 ventral primary ramus

36. A builder is brought into A&E following a fall from a ladder. He was knocked unconscious, and has a suspected facial fracture, so is sent for a CT scan.

    In the image below, what term best describes the structure indicated by the arrow?

    (a) Frontal sinus
    (b) Ethmoidal sinus
    (c) Maxillary sinus
    (d) Nasal cavity
    (e) Sphenoidal sinus

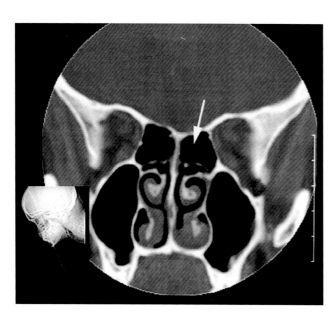

37. A child is brought into A&E with a mid-shaft fracture of the humerus following a fall from a tree.

    Which of the following structures is most at risk of damage from this injury?

    (a) Axillary nerve
    (b) Median nerve
    (c) Musculocutaneous nerve
    (d) Radial nerve
    (e) Ulnar nerve

38. A 22-year-old-man is brought into A&E following a fall from a motorbike. He has pain and swelling round his right elbow, and an X-ray reveals a fracture involving the medial epicondyle.

    What term best describes the muscles that attach at this point?

    (a) Extensors of the fingers and thumb
    (b) Extensors of the wrist
    (c) Flexors of the elbow
    (d) Flexors of the fingers and wrist
    (e) Supinators of the forearm

39. While training for a boxing match, a young athlete punches a bit too hard and dislocates the fifth metacarpophalangeal joint of his left hand.

    Which of the following terms best describes the metacarpophalangeal joints?

    (a) Ball and socket
    (b) Condylar
    (c) Hinge
    (d) Pivot
    (e) Saddle

40. After a fall onto her outstretched left hand, a 60-year-old woman is sent for an X-ray (shown below).

    Identify the structure indicated by the arrow.

    (a) Capitate
    (b) Hamate
    (c) Scaphoid
    (d) Trapezium
    (e) Trapezoid

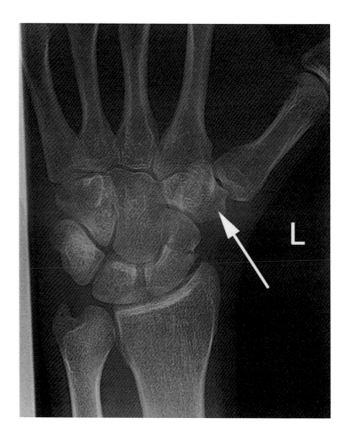

41. An obese man collapses on the street and is brought into A&E. The SHO makes an emergency incision one finger's breadth anterior to the medial malleolus in order to gain access to a blood vessel.

    What term best describes the vascular structure found at this location?

    (a) Anterior tibial artey
    (b) Femoral artery
    (c) Great saphenous vein
    (d) Posterior tibial artery
    (e) Short saphenous vein

42. In carrying out a physical examination of a patient's chest you palpate the manubriosternal joint.

    What statement best describes the vertebral level of this joint?

    (a) It is at the level of the C7/T1 vertebral disc
    (b) It is at the level of the T1/T2 vertebral disc
    (c) It is at the level of the T4/T5 vertebral disc
    (d) It is at the level of the T6/T7 vertebral disc
    (e) It is at the level of the T12/L1 vertebral disc

43. While carrying out an assessment of a coma patient, you press firmly on the medial part of the superior margin of the orbit.

    What term best describes the nerve that emerges at this point?

    (a) Frontal nerve
    (b) Infraorbital nerve
    (c) Supraorbital nerve
    (d) Temporal division of the facial nerve
    (e) Zygomatic division of the facial nerve

44. Following a blow to the head, a 40-year-old man is sent for a skull X-ray (shown below).

    From the list below, which muscle has its superior attachment at the point indicated by the arrow?

    (a) Masseter
    (b) Mylohyoid
    (c) Scalenus anterior
    (d) Sternocleidomastoid
    (e) Temporalis

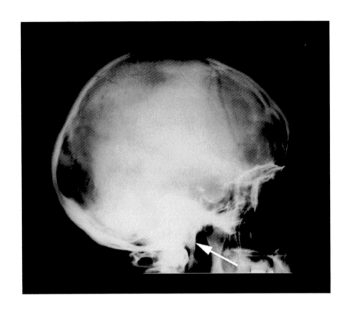

ANSWERS

1. (a)	23. (a)
2. (c)	24. (a)
3. (e)	25. (a)
4. (a)	26. (a)
5. (c)	27. (d)
6. (d)	28. (e)
7. (c)	29. (d)
8. (a)	30. (a)
9. (c)	31. (d)
10. (a)	32. (d)
11. (d)	33. (c)
12. (e)	34. (c)
13. (a)	35. (b)
14. (a)	36. (b)
15. (e)	37. (d)
16. (d)	38. (d)
17. (e)	39. (b)
18. (b)	40. (d)
19. (d)	41. (c)
20. (d)	42. (c)
21. (e)	43. (c)
22. (e)	44. (d)

7 Test yourself! Colouring images
Somayyeh Shahsavari

UPPER LIMB

1._____
2._____
3._____
4._____
5._____
6._____

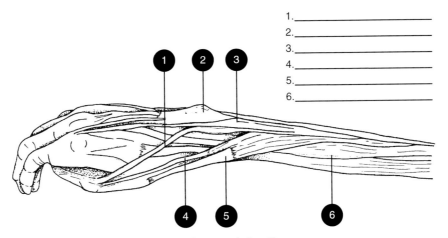

Figure 1 The anatomical snuffbox.

1._____   6._____
2._____   7._____
3._____   8._____
4._____   9._____
5._____   10._____

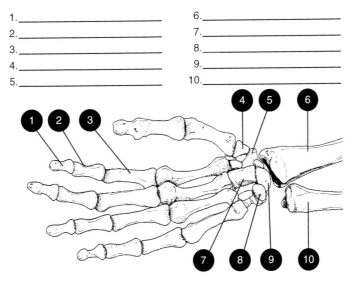

Figure 2 Bones of the hand.

1._____   5._____
2._____   6._____
3._____   7._____
4._____

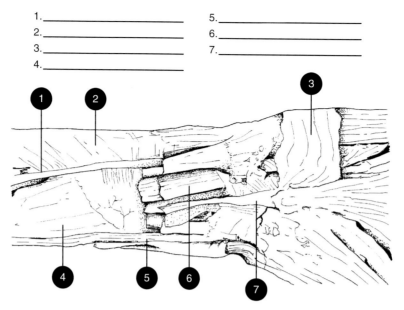

Figure 3 Anterior forearm; the wrist.

1._____
2._____
3._____
4._____

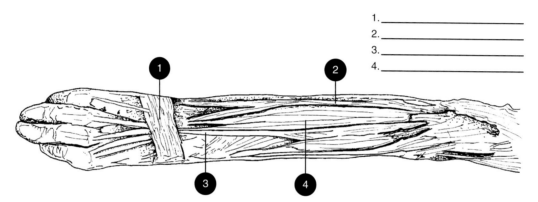

Figure 4 Posterior forearm.

1._____
2._____
3._____
4._____

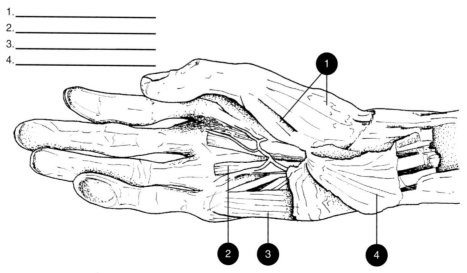

Figure 5a Hand eminences.

1._____
2._____
3._____
4._____
5._____
6._____
7._____

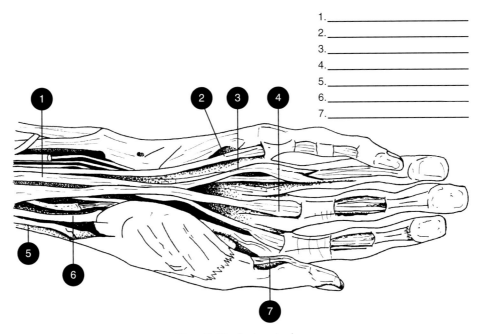

Figure 5b Hand palmar tendons.

1._____   4._____
2._____   5._____
3._____   6._____

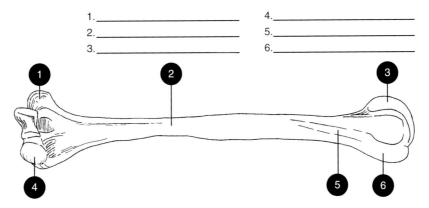

Figure 6a Humerus (anterior).

1._____
2._____
3._____
4._____

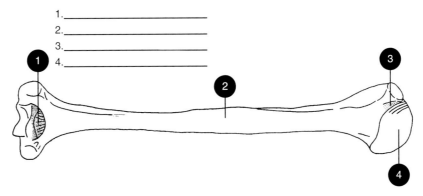

Figure 6b Humerus (posterior).

1._____   5._____
2._____   6._____
3._____   7._____
4._____   8._____

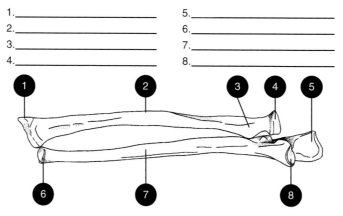

Figure 7 Forearm.

1._____
2._____
3._____
4._____
5._____
6._____
7._____

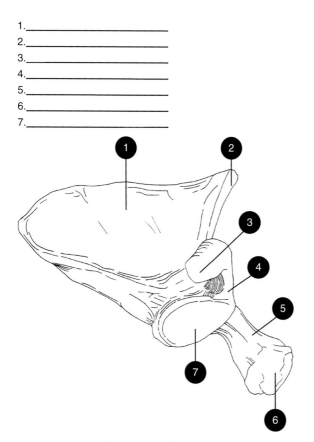

Figure 8a Scapula anterior.

1._____
2._____
3._____
4._____
5._____
6._____
7._____

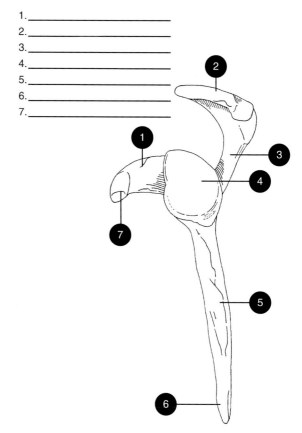

Figure 8b Scapula lateral.

1._____
2._____
3._____

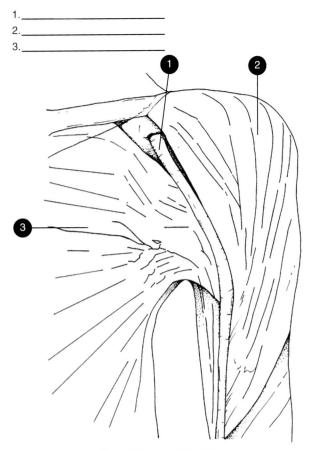

Figure 9 Upper arm/shoulder.

LOWER LIMB

1._____
2._____
3._____
4._____
5._____
6._____
7._____
8._____

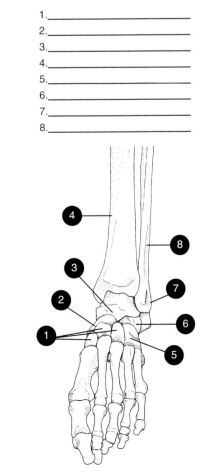

Figure 10a Foot anterior.

1._____   4._____
2._____   5._____
3._____   6._____

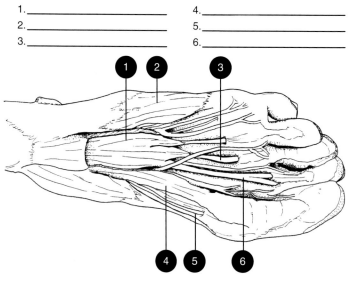

Figure 10b Foot: plantar aspect, superficial.

1._____   5._____
2._____   6._____
3._____   7._____
4._____

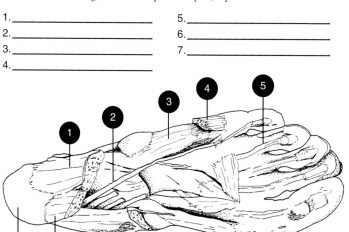

Figure 10c Foot: plantar aspect, deep.

1._____
2._____
3._____
4._____
5._____
6._____
7._____
8._____
9._____
10._____
11._____
12._____

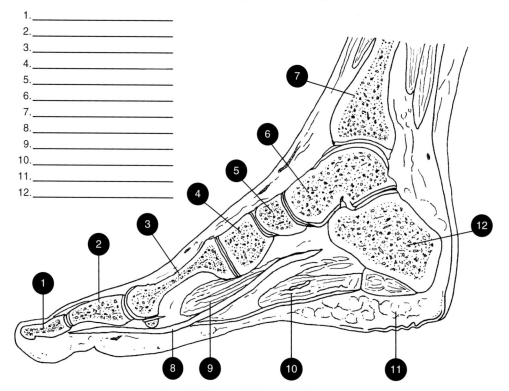

Figure 10d Bones of the foot, sagittal section.

1._____
2._____
3._____
4._____
5._____
6._____
7._____

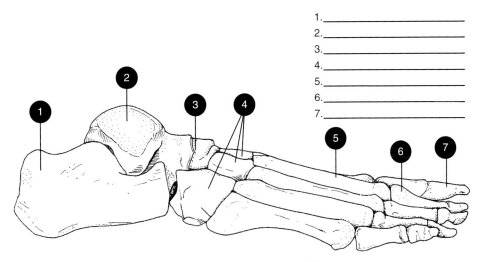

Figure 10e Bones of the foot (lateral).

1._____	5._____
2._____	6._____
3._____	7._____
4._____	8._____

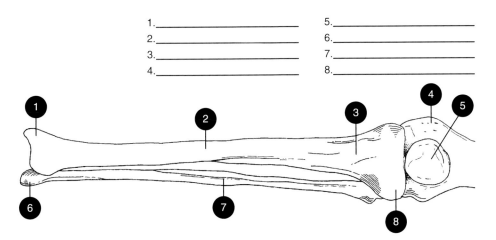

Figure 11a Leg: Tibia, fibula, patella.

1._____	5._____
2._____	6._____
3._____	7._____
4._____	

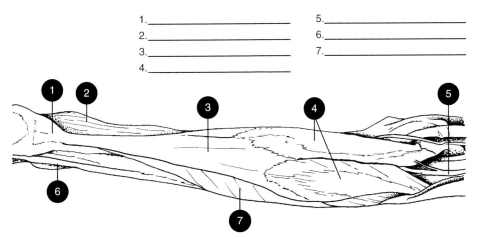

Figure 11b Leg posterior.

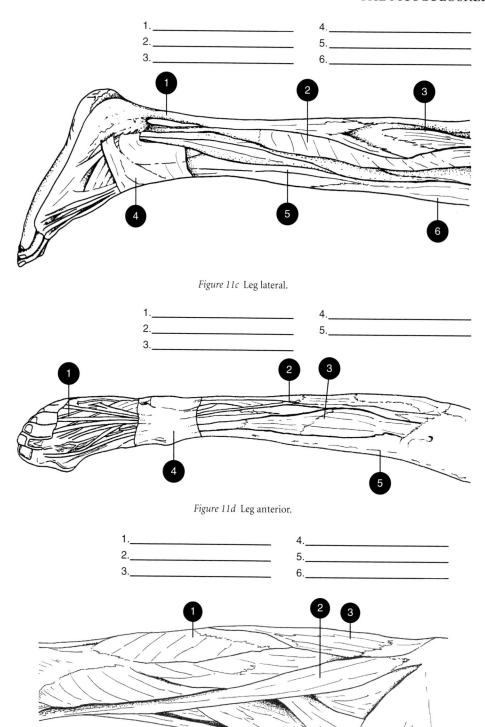

1._____   4._____
2._____   5._____
3._____   6._____

Figure 11c Leg lateral.

1._____   4._____
2._____   5._____
3._____

Figure 11d Leg anterior.

1._____   4._____
2._____   5._____
3._____   6._____

Figure 12a Thigh anterior.

1._____   4._____
2._____   5._____
3._____   6._____

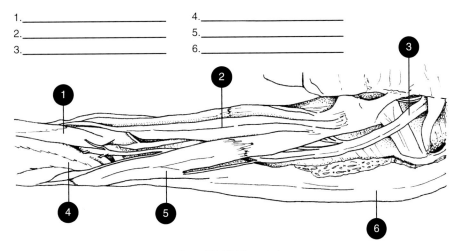

Figure 12b Thigh posterior.

1._____   6._____
2._____   7._____
3._____   8._____
4._____   9._____
5._____   10._____

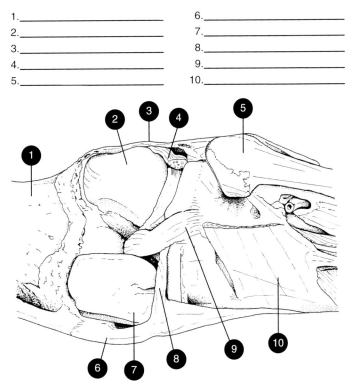

Figure 13 Knee posterior.

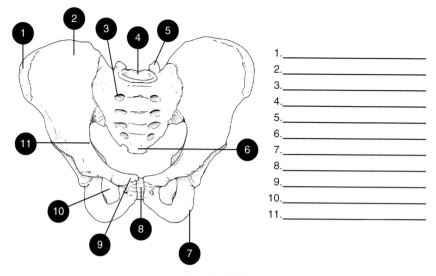

1._____
2._____
3._____
4._____
5._____
6._____
7._____
8._____
9._____
10._____
11._____

Figure 14a Pelvis.

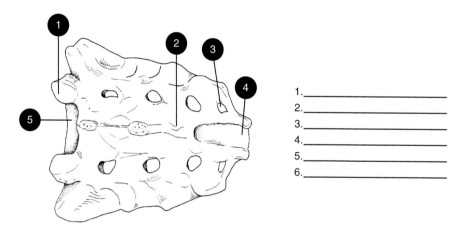

1._____
2._____
3._____
4._____
5._____
6._____

Figure 14b Sacrum, posterior.

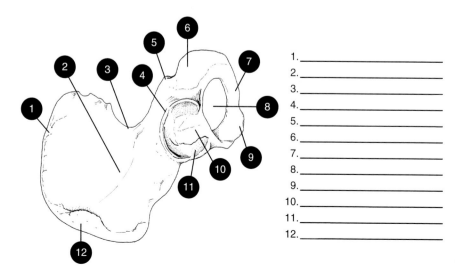

1._____
2._____
3._____
4._____
5._____
6._____
7._____
8._____
9._____
10._____
11._____
12._____

Figure 14c Pelvis lateral.

(A)

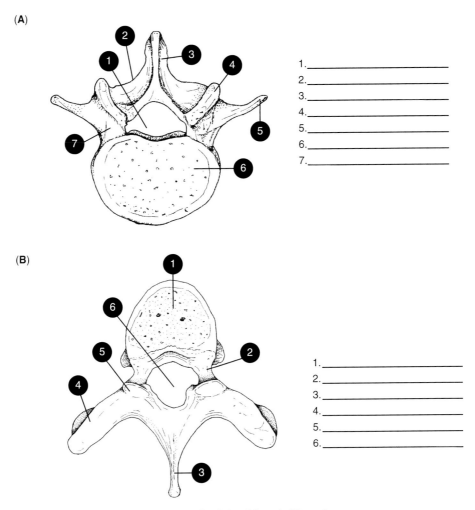

1._____
2._____
3._____
4._____
5._____
6._____
7._____

(B)

1._____
2._____
3._____
4._____
5._____
6._____

Figure 15 Lumbar (**A**) and thoracic (**B**) vertebrae.

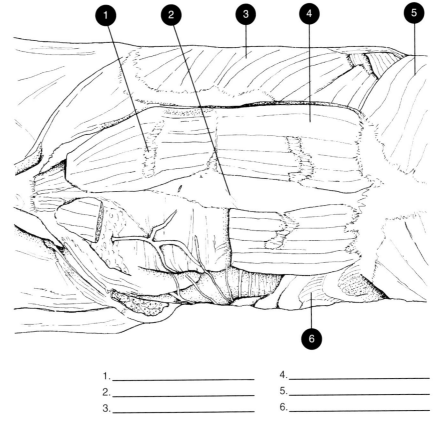

1._____   4._____
2._____   5._____
3._____   6._____

Figure 16 Abdomen.

(A)

(B)

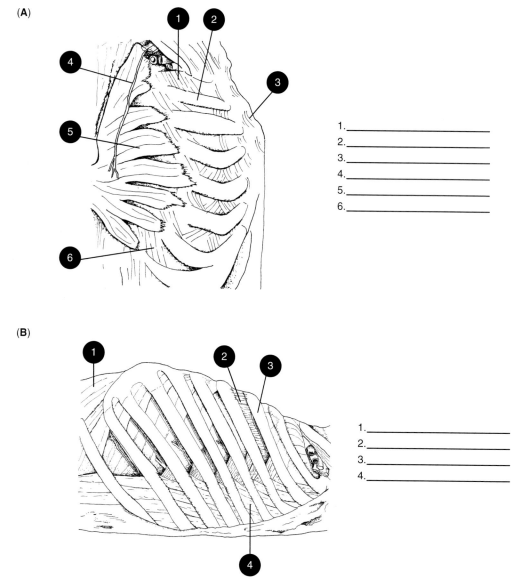

1._____
2._____
3._____
4._____
5._____
6._____

1._____
2._____
3._____
4._____

Figure 17 (**A**, **B**) Thorax.

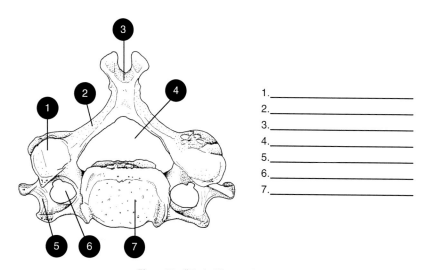

1._____
2._____
3._____
4._____
5._____
6._____
7._____

Figure 18a "Typical" cervical vertebra.

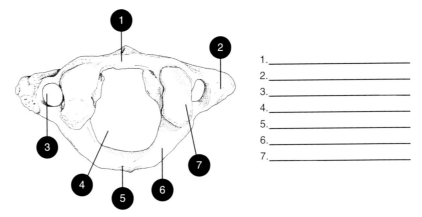

1._____
2._____
3._____
4._____
5._____
6._____
7._____

Figure 18b Cervical vertebrae C1 (atlas).

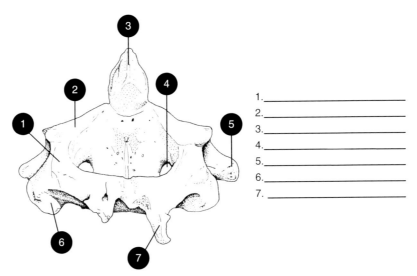

1._____
2._____
3._____
4._____
5._____
6._____
7._____

Figure 18c Cervical vertebrae C2 (axis).

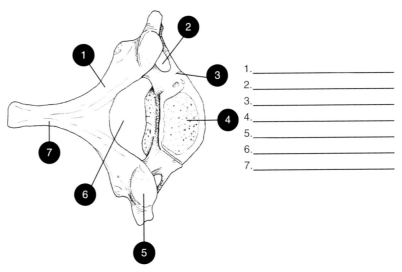

1._____
2._____
3._____
4._____
5._____
6._____
7._____

Figure 18d 7th Cervical vertebra (*vertebra prominens*)

1._____
2._____
3._____
4._____
5._____

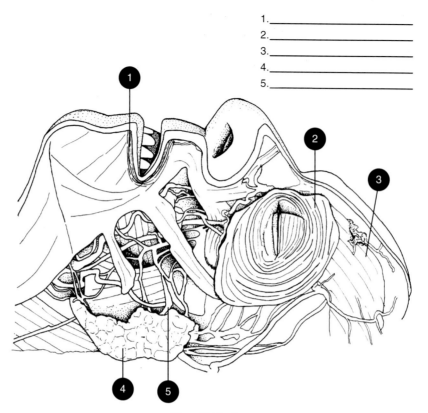

Figure 19 The face.

1._____
2._____
3._____
4._____
5._____
6._____

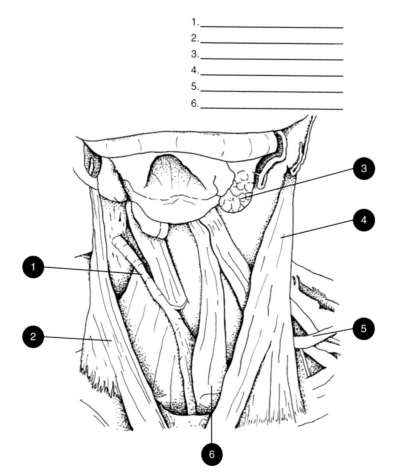

Figure 20 Anterior neck.

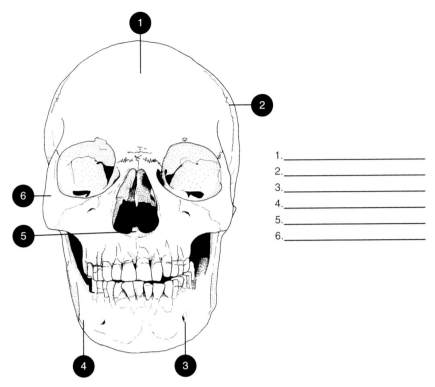

1. _____
2. _____
3. _____
4. _____
5. _____
6. _____

Figure 21a Skull anterior.

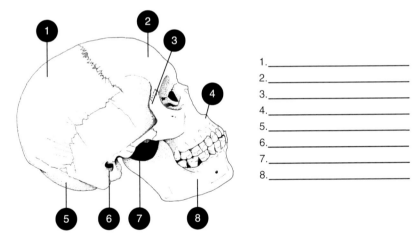

1. _____
2. _____
3. _____
4. _____
5. _____
6. _____
7. _____
8. _____

Figure 21b Skull lateral.

Index

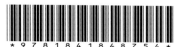

T - #1060 - 101024 - C136 - 285/214/6 [8] - CB - 9781841848754 - Gloss Lamination